S0-AAF-140

FORGOTTEN PEOPLE, FORGOTTEN DISEASES

FORGOTTEN PEOPLE, FORGOTTEN DISEASES

The Neglected Tropical Diseases and Their Impact on Global Health and Development

Peter J. Hotez, M.D., Ph.D.

The George Washington University
and
Sabin Vaccine Institute
Washington, DC

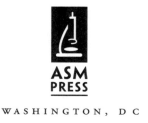

ASM
PRESS

WASHINGTON, DC

Cover art: "A Ray of Hope" by Emma Burns (from PLoS NTDs, Oct. 2007, vol. 1, no. 1), depicting the darkness of disease contrasted with the light and hope that scientific research brings to global health and wellness.

Copyright © 2008 ASM Press
      American Society for Microbiology
      1752 N Street, N.W.
      Washington, DC 20036-2904

Library of Congress Cataloging-in-Publication Data

Hotez, Peter J.
  Forgotten people, forgotten diseases : the neglected tropical diseases and their impact on global health and development / Peter J. Hotez.
    p. ; cm.
  Includes bibliographical references and index.
  ISBN 978-1-55581-440-3
  1. Tropical medicine. I. Title.
  [DNLM: 1. Parasitic Diseases—prevention & control. 2. Antiparasitic Agents—therapeutic use. 3. Developing Countries—economics. 4. International Cooperation. 5. Tropical Medicine. 6. World Health. WC 695 H832f 2008]

  RC961.H68 2008
  362.196′9883—dc22
                                   2008010700

All Rights Reserved
Printed in the United States of America

10 9 8 7 6 5 4 3 2 1

Address editorial correspondence to: ASM Press, 1752 N St., N.W., Washington, DC 20036-2904, U.S.A.

Send orders to: ASM Press, P.O. Box 605, Herndon, VA 20172, U.S.A.
Phone: 800-546-2416; 703-661-1593
Fax: 703-661-1501
Email: Books@asmusa.org
Online: estore.asm.org

Dedicated to my youngest daughter,
Rachel Kate Hotez,
who teaches me every day about disabilities

To the memory of my brother,
Richard Eric Hotes, M.D.

And to the Bill and Melinda Gates Foundation
for the opportunity to devote my
life to the Neglected Tropical Diseases

Contents

Foreword

Like a great general mustering his forces, Prof. Peter Hotez is gathering the forces of the world community to the fight against mankind's most ancient scourges: leprosy, worm infections, blinding trachoma, and other harrowing tropical diseases. Hotez is an able leader in this great battle. His crystal clear and powerful text displays the mind of a great scientist and humanist, one who knows every technical detail about the diseases which afflict billions of people and kill millions each decade. But Hotez never overlooks the afflicted themselves, the poor people of Africa, Asia, and Latin America among whom he's worked throughout his path-breaking career. Most importantly of all, he provides not only facts but also solutions, how we can finally triumph in an age-old struggle by deploying the best of modern public health and medical science.

In recent years, Hotez and several other world leaders in public health, including David Molyneux (Liverpool School of Medicine), Alan Fenwick (Imperial College London), and Lorenzo Savioli (World Health Organization), have been alerting the world to new possibilities to confront crippling diseases that have been long out of the limelight—indeed, often stigmatized to the point of systematic neglect, but taking a huge and devastating toll nonetheless. These leaders have christened these diseases the Neglected Tropical Diseases, or NTDs, and, in a crusade that combines elegant science with public education on a global scale, have created a new awareness of the possibility of making decisive advances in disease control. In essence, Hotez aims to take the "N" out of NTDs and to replace it with an "F," so that these become the Former Tropical Diseases, at least in the sense of being brought decisively under control if not fully eliminated.

This book is an amazing and invaluable primer. It can be read by the general reader but also by the Infectious Diseases specialist. The general reader will no doubt feel stretched by the countless disease pathways, pathogenic agents, types of controls, and variations around the world. Yet at the same time, the reader will feel exhilarated by seeing this complex and fascinating world presented with the utmost clarity, historical insight, and optimism. For this is a tale not only of harrowing suffering, but also of largely, and sometimes wholly, remediable suffering. As shocking and devastating are some of the stories, figures, and pictures, there is no gloom, only the steely determination to do all that we can as a global society to get these diseases under control.

The book is organized in a compelling manner. After a powerful overview showing that these diseases, despite their relative neglect, carry a combined disease burden on the same order of magnitude as AIDS, tuberculosis, and malaria, Hotez takes us on a remarkable tour of the world of worms and other pathogens, the disease vectors (such as mosquitoes and flies) which transmit them, and the state of public health and medical science. The agenda is daunting, with no fewer than thirteen killers playing a leading role and countless lesser infections also making cameo appearances. Yet the writing is so clear and compelling that, instead of jumble, Hotez provides us with an intellectual framework to keep the big picture even as we tour the water holes, lymph nodes, intestines, and mosquito salivary glands which constitute the settings of Hotez's dramatic stories.

After explaining clearly and compellingly, but never condescendingly, the complexities of these tropical infections—including the pathogens which cause them, their transmission routes, the links to poverty, the pharmacology, and the history of control methods, right up to the present—Hotez rounds off the text with four crucial chapters. In chapter 9 he reminds us, forcefully but not alarmingly, that these are not only diseases of the tropical nations but also of the United States (at least in some cases). We have to care, not only for what these diseases mean for global suffering and for global political stability, but also for what they mean right at home in the U.S. In chapter 10 he describes the heroic efforts of many leaders, such as former President Jimmy Carter, and countless organizations and the new hopes for a stronger global leadership pulled together by a new Global Network for NTD Control, an effort in which Hotez has played a decisive role. In chapter 11 he reminds us that all effective public health programs, including the comprehensive control of the NTDs, must combine the comprehensive use of our existing tools—medicines, bed nets, surveillance, and others—with the research and development of new and more powerful tools, including vaccines against many of the NTDs. Characteristically, Hotez himself is a pioneer in research and development of a hookworm vaccine.

In the closing chapter 12, Hotez again raises the stakes. Controlling the NTDs is nothing less than "healing the world." The control of the NTDs is a matter not only of disease control, but also of global security. Hotez argues persuasively that the NTDs, together with other killers such as AIDS, tuberculosis, and malaria, not only are exacerbated by upheavals of violence and conflict, but also are causes of conflict through their devastating effects of poverty, hunger, and despair, all precursors to violence in the poorest countries.

This book is thrilling on all levels. It is a unique opportunity for a wide readership to understand the science behind many of the world's leading afflictions.

It is an opportunity to draw hope from countless examples of how science is contributing to solutions and the chances for comprehensive control of these killer diseases. And it is an invitation to all of us to engage personally with one of the greatest challenges of our time: using our heads and our hearts to help solve some of the longest-standing scourges facing humanity, and thereby building a world of greater justice, shared prosperity, and security.

Sonia Ehrlich Sachs, M.D., M.P.H.
Coordinator of Public Health Programs
Millennium Village Project of The Earth Institute
Columbia University, New York, New York

Jeffrey D. Sachs, Ph.D.
Special Advisor to UN Secretary General Ban Ki-Moon
Director of The Earth Institute
Columbia University, New York, New York

Foreword

In my humanitarian missions to Angola and elsewhere in developing countries, I am always struck by the devastation wrought by disease and malnutrition. Watching children and young women fall ill or fail to reach their full potential because of circumstances beyond their control has imprinted many indelible images in my mind. Although I have tried to capture some of this human suffering in my black and white photography, I also know there is so much more hidden misery that cannot be captured through pictures.

In my role as Lead Ambassador for the Global Network for Neglected Tropical Diseases, I have learned firsthand about the largely silent suffering that results from these terrible afflictions. Hookworms rob children of their daily iron and protein requirements and prevent them from growing and learning. Elephantiasis, Buruli ulcer, and leprosy cause disfigurement. River blindness and trachoma cause permanent vision loss. African sleeping sickness results in a slow and agonizing death.

Forgotten People, Forgotten Diseases explains in straightforward language where these neglected tropical diseases occur and how they have become the most common diseases among the world's poorest people. It also highlights the chronic and debilitating aspects of these diseases and their poverty-promoting features. Of particular importance to me, the book illustrates how people afflicted with neglected tropical diseases suffer from stigma in their communities, especially young women, who are often abandoned by their husbands and prevented from holding their children. Portrayed here is human suffering on an almost unimaginable scale.

Finally, *Forgotten People, Forgotten Diseases* teaches us about an incredible opportunity we have to control these neglected tropical diseases on a massive scale, with both existing drugs and new vaccines being developed in nonprofit research laboratories. I am excited by the possibility of witnessing the elimination of some of these terrible scourges in my lifetime. For all of these reasons, I am hopeful that this book will inspire you and stimulate you to get involved in stamping out the neglected tropical diseases, thereby taking an important step to reaching out in a very tangible way to the world's poorest and most vulnerable people.

Alyssa Milano
Lead Ambassador, Global Network for Neglected Tropical Diseases

Preface

Ever since junior high school, I have been fascinated by the application of scientific knowledge for solving tropical public health problems of global importance. Starting with an M.D.-Ph.D. dissertation begun in 1980, my adult life has been a quest to develop experimental vaccines for human hookworm infection. Now, after more than 25 years of laboratory investigation and thanks to the support of the Bill and Melinda Gates Foundation, I have the opportunity and good fortune to head a multidisciplinary team that is developing and manufacturing these vaccines and then testing them in an area of Brazil where hookworm is endemic. While reaching this goal has been intensely satisfying at both a professional and personal level, I have also come to realize that completing early-stage development of a new product for a disease such as hookworm has in many ways been the easy part! Hookworm infects approximately 600 million people worldwide, but they almost all live on less than US$2 per day and only in the poorest regions of sub-Saharan Africa, Asia, and the tropical regions of the Americas. Because the people at risk for hookworm infection cannot afford to pay for a vaccine, unless there is greater general awareness about the public health and economic importance of hookworm and other parasitic infections there will never be the political will and large-scale financial investment necessary to ensure the global access of a hookworm vaccine, or indeed any other product for the diseases of poverty. Simultaneously, as it becomes evident to me that vaccine development is a decades-long process, I feel a need to do more in order to reach out to the world's poor and provide them with better access to the existing treatments for hookworm, even if our currently available anti-hookworm drugs are imperfect.

Partly as a means to increase access to essential medicines and innovation, I have begun a concerted effort to raise public awareness of hookworm and other parasitic infections and to advocate for the largely voiceless poor people living in remote and rural regions of endemicity. However, it was only after I met three scientific "soul mates," medical parasitologists who were simultaneously launching their own advocacy efforts, that I felt an important breakthrough was achieved in terms of placing parasitic diseases on the global radar screen. Since 2003 I have engaged in intense colloquy with Professor David H. Molyneux of the Liverpool School of Tropical Medicine (David is also the Director of the Global Alliance to Eliminate Lymphatic Filariasis), Professor Alan Fenwick from Imperial College, London (Alan is also the Director of the Schistosomiasis Control Initiative), and Dr. Lorenzo Savioli from the World Health Organization (as well as some of his close colleagues there, including Drs. Denis Daumerie, Dirk Engels, and Jean Jannin) about some of the common features of all parasitic infections affecting poor people. During these long and detailed but also joyful conversations, which took place in Washington, DC, Atlanta, New York, London, Liverpool, Glasgow, Geneva, Berlin, and Stockholm, we soon realized that the major parasitic infections, as well as some selected bacterial and viral infections, could be thought of in aggregate as a group under the banner of the neglected tropical diseases, or NTDs for short. The NTDs are the most common infections of poor people, and also among the most important in terms of their health and economic impact. In many respects, their burden of disease rivals those of better-known conditions including HIV/AIDS, even though most people have never heard about the NTDs. This lack of recognition continues to surprise us given that the NTDs are ancient conditions that have plagued humankind for centuries (as documented in many of our earliest writings such as Egyptian medical papyri and religious texts, including the Bible), and they represent one of the most important reasons why the populations living in low-income countries of Africa, Asia, and Central and South America remain mired in a vicious cycle of poverty, destitution, and despair. The continued presence of NTDs in North America represents that region's most striking health disparity and a sad legacy of the Middle Passage, the Atlantic slave trade between the 15th and 19th centuries.

Professor Jeffrey Sachs and Dr. Sonia Ehrlich Sachs of Columbia's Earth Institute and Dr. Eric Ottesen (then at Emory University) subsequently joined our informal NTD working group, and in a series of policy papers published in PLoS (Public Library of Science) and the *New England Journal of Medicine*, we were able to articulate the concept of the NTDs and how we can control or eliminate them through a global scale-up of access to essential medicines. These policy documents also provided a rationale for us to establish a new Global Network for NTDs, which is working to coordinate global advocacy and resource mobilization efforts for these conditions.

Forgotten People, Forgotten Diseases summarizes in mostly nontechnical language the major concepts about the NTDs and how they cause human suffering, as well as their global importance and the unique and unusual opportunity we now have to lift the world's poorest people out of poverty through low-cost and highly cost-effective control measures.

Peter Hotez
Washington, DC

Acknowledgments

The idea for this book's title came from a 2002 paper on helminth infections written by David Crompton and Michael Nesheim in the *Annual Review of Nutrition*, in which they quoted the phrase "forgotten diseases of forgotten people" (attributed to M. G. Schultz). I was inspired to write an "NTD Manifesto" in part from Jeff Sachs's success in educating the general public about poverty in low-income countries in his landmark book, *The End of Poverty*, and also because of a very accessible book entitled *Essentials of Global Health*, written by my friend and colleague Richard Skolnik.

In addition to the individuals mentioned above and in the Preface, there are also many others who inspired me to write this book. They include my colleagues from the Global Network, including my associates at the Sabin Vaccine Institute, Kari Stoever (who provided leadership in helping to launch the Global Network, as well as her "A team"), Azalea Kim, Karen Palacio, Colin Burke, and Lindsay Wheeler; Kathy Spahn and Chad MacArthur from Helen Keller International; Jacob Kumaresan and Ibrahim Jabr from the International Trachoma Initiative; Mark Rosenberg, Eric Ottesen, and Nana Twum-Danso from the Task Force for Child Survival and Development; Joanna Rubinstein and Josh Ruxun from the Earth Institute at Columbia University; and John McCullough from Liverpool Associates in Tropical Health. I also want to acknowledge the leadership of the WHO, including Margaret Chan (Director-General), Anarfi Asamaoah Baah (Deputy Director-General), and David Heymann (Assistant Director-General, Communicable Diseases); the leadership of the Carter Center, including Donald Hopkins, Frank O. Richards, and former President Jimmy Carter and Rosalynn Carter; the Division of Parasitic Diseases of the CDC; Marcel Tanner, Juerg Utzinger, and Jennifer Kaiser at the Swiss Tropical Institute; Michael Katz at the March of Dimes Birth Defects Foundation; and Mirta Roses Periago, Director-General, Steven Ault, and the NTD group at the Pan American Health Organization for their exemplary dedication to NTDs, as well as the leadership at Merck & Co., Pfizer Inc., GlaxoSmithKline, Johnson

& Johnson, Novartis, Merck KgaA, Med Pharm, and Sanofi-Aventis for donating NTD drugs to the world. Sandeep Kishore and Prabhjot Dhadialla, two M.D.-Ph.D. students at the Weil Cornell Medical College and Rockefeller University, and Rajesh Gupta, a Stanford medical student, have helped to launch an important student-led campaign to tackle the NTDs. I wish to acknowledge with deep gratitude and respect my former mentors from Yale and Rockefeller Universities and the Massachusetts General Hospital: Curtis Patton, Frank F. Richards, George Miller, Anthony Cerami, and Jose Ignacio Santos.

Of enormous importance to the NTD enterprise is the Sabin Vaccine Institute Board Chairman, Philip K. Russell, who is my very important mentor on all things vaccines and global health, as well as his wife, Connie Russell. Ciro de Quadros, one of the giants of vaccinology and global health, has also been a source of inspiration and much-needed advice and wisdom. I also want to extend my deepest appreciation to my close friends and colleagues at the Human Hookworm Vaccine Initiative (HHVI) based at the Sabin Vaccine Institute, H. R. Shepherd, the Founding Chair, and his wife, Carol Ruth; Heloisa Sabin; Mort and Chris Hyman for their particular commitment to NTDs and their very important early support for schistosmiasis vaccine development; and to the rest of the Sabin Board members: Mary Ann Chaffee, Lou Cooper, Brian Davis, Jeffrey Fuisz, Lance Gordon, Nancy Gardner Hargrave, Axel Hoos, Michael and Jacqueline Kempner, Clark McFadden, Walter Orenstein, Ciro de Quadros, Kevin L. Reilly, Adan Rios, and Michael Whitham. I acknowledge the support of some very important people at The George Washington University Medical Center, including Jim Scott, Allan Goldstein, Richard Skolnik, Richard Southby, Ruth Katz, George Davis, Victor Barbiero, Gary Simon, Alan Wasserman, and John F. "Skip" Williams, past GWU President Stephen Joel Trachtenberg, and the new GWU president, Steven Knapp.

I want to thank my close scientific colleagues and friends at the HHVI, including Jeff Bethony, Maria Elena Bottazzi, Simon Brooker, Ami Shah Brown, David Diemert, Ricardo Fujiwara, Gaddam Narsa Goud, Kathryn Jones, Alex Loukas, Beth Martins, Rodrigo Correa Oliveira, Isaias Raw, Helton Santiago, Peter Smith, and Bin Zhan, as well as Vehid Deumic, Richi Gupta, Desheng Jiang, Brian Keegan, Patti Lieblich, Aaron Miles, Julie Ost, Jordan Plieskatt, Tracey Smith, Irene Thuo, Weston Williams, Nate Wolf, and Sharon Wu. Sophia Raff and Tania Govanlu were especially helpful in working with me to prepare the manuscripts for this book. A special thanks to Sophia Chung-Debose. The outstanding staff at *PLoS Neglected Tropical Diseases*, including Gavin Yamey, Dan Sarna, and Shab Sigman, and the leadership at PLoS, including Harold Varmus, represent important individuals in our NTD advocacy efforts. The open-access neglected disease series of papers from *PLoS Medicine* were extremely useful and authoritative references and provided many of the figures for this book, as did the Public Health Image Library of the CDC.

I want to express deepest gratitude to the program officers of the Gates Foundation, who advocated for us and made it possible for me to pursue a dream and have a career devoted to hookworm vaccine development and NTD control. They include David Brandling-Bennett, Julie Jacobson, Gordon Perkin,

Gina Rabinovich, Tadataka Yamada, and Gabrielle Fitzgerald. I am especially grateful for the active and personal involvement of Bill and Melinda Gates.

I am deeply appreciative of my good colleagues at Geneva Global and Legatum for rolling the dice with us on the scale-up of NTD control, and John Robbins at the NIH for all his advice and support. In addition, former President William Jefferson Clinton, Senator Hillary Rodham Clinton, and the outstanding staff of the Clinton Global Initiative (including Tom Kalil, Chris Jennings, and Sara Richlin) have lent a powerful voice to NTDs. Senators Sam Brownback, John Kerry, and Edward Kennedy and their staffs have also made the NTDs a major priority.

Based on his personal experiences in the Democratic Republic of Congo and elsewhere in developing countries, Dikembe Mutombo of the Houston Rockets has been a powerful force behind the movement to raise awareness of the NTDs. I also thank the comedian Jill-Michele Meleán.

Beloved everywhere, Alyssa Milano, our Global Network for NTDs Ambassador, has given a fresh and beautiful face to these conditions and new hope to people everywhere who suffer from the stigma and disfigurement of the NTDs. She has been an eloquent and passionate spokesperson for these conditions.

Finally, I want to thank my loving family, Ann, Matthew, Emy, Rachel, and Daniel Hotez, as well as Larry and Linda Hotes, Liz and Warren Kirshenbaum, Andrea Hotes, and parents Ed and Jean Hotez; nephews and nieces Gennifer, Josh, Todd, Andrew, Alyssa, Marissa, Sammy, and Julia; in-laws Don, Marsha, Julia, and David Frifield, Mark and Judy Conway, and Irv and Peggy Goldberg; Daniel and Nancy Goldberg and their families, and all of the others in my extended family and circle of friends for putting up with me all of these years!

chapter 1

Introduction to the Neglected Tropical Diseases

The age of hypocrisy has been succeeded by that of indifference, which is worse, for indifference corrupts and appeases: it kills the spirit before it kills the body. It has been stated before, it bears repeating: the opposite of love is not hate, but indifference.

ELIE WIESEL, *A JEW TODAY*

It is a trite saying that one half the world knows not how the other lives. Who can say what sores might be healed, what hurts solved, were the doings of each half of the world's inhabitants understood and appreciated by the other?

MAHATMA GANDHI

During this first decade of the 21st century, we have seen unfold a new sense of urgency about the plight of the world's poorest people in developing countries. Today, the average well-educated layperson living in "the North" (North America, Europe, and Japan) is far more aware than ever before about the suffering of the people living in "the South" (the developing countries of sub-Saharan Africa, Asia, and the Americas). Almost certainly, the human catastrophe of HIV/AIDS in sub-Saharan Africa, known as the "plague of the 21st century," and concerns about possible pandemics from influenza and SARS have helped to focus world attention on health problems in developing countries.[1] Simultaneously, an unprecedented and extraordinary advocacy effort led by some highly influential international leaders and celebrities has helped to fuel a 21st-century global health movement. Bono, Angelina Jolie, Brad Pitt, Bill and Melinda Gates, Jeffrey Sachs, Oprah Winfrey, Bob Geldof, Tony Blair, Jimmy Carter, and Bill Clinton have donated their time and energy to advocate for the health of the world's poorest people. These efforts have captivated world attention and have even infused an element of glamor into solving global health problems. Between 2005 and 2006 alone, Bono, Bill Gates, and Melinda Gates were named *Time* magazine Persons of the Year; the Time Global Health Summit in New York was branded the "Woodstock of global health"; Brad Pitt narrated a 6-h-long documentary, "Rx for Survival, a Global Health Challenge," for PBS; former President Clinton featured global health issues at his annual Clinton Global Initiative; and Bono and Bobby Shriver launched Product RED to support HIV/AIDS, malaria, and tuberculosis relief at the 2006 World Economic Forum in Davos, Switzerland.[2] As a professor, I can attest that these activities stimulated an unprecedented level of interest in global health issues from both undergraduates and graduate public health and medical students. These days, almost every week during the academic year, I am visited by one or more young persons who request advice on how they can help solve a health problem in a developing country. I am not the only faculty member to have this experience—today, new university-wide global health institutes are springing up at Duke, Vanderbilt, Harvard, Emory, University of Washington, and elsewhere, as university deans and presidents scramble to keep up with student interest.

Like any movement, the one in global health has been stimulated by a manifesto, defined by Webster as "a public declaration of motives and intentions by a government or by a person or group regarded as having some public importance."[1] For the global health movement, we can point to at least three landmark 21st-century policy documents, which have effectively served as manifestos.

The first of these documents had its origins in January 2000, when then WHO Director-General Gro Harlem Brundtland launched the Commission on Macroeconomics and Health (CMH) and appointed the international macroeconomist Jeffrey Sachs to serve as its chair. Jeff and his colleagues were charged with analyzing the impact of health on development, and their *Report of the CMH*, which was illustrated with examples of how health investments translate into economic development, elegantly articulated a profound relationship between disease and chronic poverty. As a result, the world's most influential finance ministers and policymakers began to regard improvements in global health as an important tool for poverty reduction. A second initiative was also launched in 2000 when the General Assembly of the UN convened in New York City in order to adopt a resolution known as the UN Millennium Declaration. The Declaration was a renewed call for sustainable development and for the eradication of poverty, and its core was a set of eight specific Millennium Development Goals (MDGs) along with a set of specific targets for the year 2015. As shown in Table 1.1, three of the goals (MDGs 4, 5, and 6) specifically emphasize health. Finally, the third manifesto was the *Report of the Commission for Africa*, commissioned by British Prime Minister Tony Blair in order to accelerate the development of Africa. The report served as an important blueprint for commitments by the Group of Eight (G8) nations at their 2005 summit in Gleneagles, Scotland.

Unlike many UN and international declarations, which too often are forgotten by the global community almost as soon as they are written, the *CMH Report*, the MDGs, and the *Report of the Commission for Africa* continue to exert a major influence on global policymakers. Equally important, together

Table 1.1 The MDGs

1.	Eradicate extreme poverty and hunger
2.	Achieve universal primary education
3.	Promote gender equality and empower women
4.	Reduce child mortality
5.	Improve maternal health
6.	Combat HIV/AIDS, malaria, and other diseases
7.	Ensure environmental sustainability
8.	Develop a global partnership for development

with the new advocacy by leaders and celebrities, the global health manifestos have stimulated high-level efforts to invent innovative financial instruments for supported disease control, including some very substantial funding initiatives from both the G8 nations and some prominent private philanthropic organizations such as the Bill and Melinda Gates Foundation.

MDG 6 ("To combat HIV/AIDS, malaria, and other diseases") has been a particular target of these new funds, with billions of dollars appropriated by the U.S. Congress for HIV/AIDS and malaria through the President's Emergency Plan for AIDS Relief (PEPFAR) and the President's Malaria Initiative (PMI), respectively. Internationally, the Global Fund to Fight AIDS, Tuberculosis, and Malaria ("The Global Fund") has so far committed US$7.1 billion in 136 countries to support interventions against these diseases, while the Gates Foundation has committed more than US$1 billion.[2] Practically speaking, these extraordinary new financial commitments mean that unprecedented numbers of poor people in Africa and elsewhere are receiving lifesaving antiretroviral medications for the treatment of HIV/AIDS or drugs and bed nets for the treatment and prevention of malaria. Such interventions are expected to make significant positive changes on the global health landscape over the coming decade.

Unfortunately, with the exception of some important support from the Gates Foundation, the flurry of global health advocacy and resource mobilization occurring over the past few years has largely bypassed the third "other diseases" component of MDG 6.[2] This neglect is particularly true for a group of exotic-sounding tropical infections that represent a health and socioeconomic problem of extraordinary dimensions but one that only now world leaders and global health advocates are recognizing. The core group of the 13 major so-called neglected tropical diseases or NTDs is listed in Table 1.2. They include the major parasitic worm infections of humans, such as ascariasis (roundworm infection), hookworm infection, trichuriasis (whipworm infection), lymphatic filariasis (LF or elephantiasis), schistosomiasis (snail fever), onchocerciasis (river blindness), and dracunculiasis (guinea worm infection); an important group of infections caused by single-celled protozoan parasites such as Chagas' disease, leishmaniasis, and human African trypanosomiasis (sleeping sickness); and some atypical bacterial infections, such as trachoma and the mycobacterial infections (Buruli ulcer and leprosy). Additional tropical infections can also be considered NTDs, and there is an expanded list of these conditions included in the appendix.

Table 1.2 The NTDs (core group of 13)

Infection type	Disease or pathogen name
Helminth (worm) infections	
STH[a] infections.	Ascariasis (roundworm)
	Hookworm infection
	Trichuriasis (whipworm)
Other helminth infections	Schistosomiasis (snail fever)
	LF (elephantiasis)
	Onchocerciasis (river blindness)
	Dracunculiasis (guinea worm)
Protozoan infections	Leishmaniasis
	Chagas' disease
	Human African trypanosomiasis
	(sleeping sickness)
Bacterial infections	Trachoma
	Buruli ulcer
	Leprosy

[a]STH, soil-transmitted helminth.

While many educated people have by now learned something about HIV/ AIDS and malaria and their impact in Africa and elsewhere in the developing world, far fewer have heard about this core group of NTDs. Therefore, it may come as a surprise to learn that the NTDs represent some of the most common infections of the world's poorest people. Today, of the 6.6 billion people living on our planet, an estimated 1 billion people live on less than US$1 per day and 2.7 billion people live on less than US$2 per day. As shown in Table 1.3, approximately one-fourth of the poorest 2.7 billion people suffer from ascariasis, trichuriasis, or hookworm infection, parasitic worm infections that are transmitted through the contaminated warm and moist soil of tropical developing countries (and are known as the "soil-transmitted helminth infections"), while roughly 1 in 10 of the world's poorest people suffers from schistosomiasis, 1 in 20 from LF and trachoma, and 1 in 50 from onchocerciasis.[3] Overall, approximately 1 billion people, almost 40% of the world's poorest people, are affected by one or more of the seven most common NTDs—ascariasis, trichuriasis, hookworm infection, schistosomiasis, LF, trachoma, and onchocerciasis.

Shown in Color Plate 1 are the countries in which five or more of these NTDs occur.[3] The extensive geographic overlap of these conditions means that many of the NTDs are *coendemic* and that it is common for poor people to be simultaneously infected with multiple NTDs. Of the 56 nations with five or more coendemic NTDs, 40 are found in Africa, nine in Asia, five in the Americas, and two in the Middle East. Today, Africa accounts for 100% of all of the world's cases of dracunculiasis, 99% of the cases of onchocerciasis, almost 90% of the world's cases of schistosomiasis, approximately 40% of the cases of LF and trachoma, and one-third of the world's hookworm infection.[4] The

Table 1.3 The 13 major NTDs ranked by prevalence[a]

Disease	Global prevalence	Population at risk	Regions of highest prevalence
Ascariasis	807 million	4.2 billion	East Asia-Pacific, sub-Saharan Africa, India and South Asia, Latin America
Trichuriasis	604 million	3.2 billion	Sub-Saharan Africa, East Asia-Pacific, Latin America, India and South Asia
Hookworm infection	576 million	3.2 billion	Sub-Saharan Africa, East Asia-Pacific, India and South Asia, Latin America
Schistosomiasis	207 million	779 million	Sub-Saharan Africa, Latin America
LF	120 million	1.3 billion	India and South Asia, sub-Saharan Africa, East Asia-Pacific
Trachoma	84 million	590 million	Sub-Saharan Africa, Middle East and North Africa South Asia, East Asia-Pacific
Onchocerciasis	37 million	90 million	Sub-Saharan Africa, Latin America
Leishmaniasis	12 million	350 million	India and South Asia, sub-Saharan Africa, Latin America
Chagas' disease	8–9 million	25 million	Latin America
Leprosy	0.4 million	ND[b]	India, sub-Saharan Africa, Latin America
Human African trypanosomiasis	0.3 million	60 million	Sub-Saharan Africa
Buruli ulcer	0.05 million	ND	Sub-Saharan Africa
Dracunculiaisis	0.01 million	ND	Sub-Saharan Africa

[a]Modified from Hotez et al., 2007b.
[b]ND, not determined.

impoverished areas of Asia, especially Southeast Asia and the Indian subcontinent, account for more than one-half of the world's cases of hookworm, ascariasis, and LF. Hookworm, schistosomiasis, LF, and onchocerciasis also remain highly endemic in focal regions of American tropics and subtropics, especially in Central America and Brazil, where it has been suggested that these NTDs represent a living legacy of the Middle Passage, the forced transportation of Africans to the Americas.[5] Today, these NTDs still primarily afflict the poor and marginalized people living in the region.[5]

In addition to their geographic overlap and coendemicity, the major NTDs exhibit a remarkable set of common features, all of which adversely affect the health and socioeconomic status of the world's poorest people (Table 1.4).[6]

To summarize these common features:

1. *High prevalence.* As discussed above, today the NTDs are among the most common infections of the poorest people in developing countries.[3]
2. *The link between NTDs and rural poverty.* The high prevalence of the NTDs is frequently not widely appreciated by policymakers or sometimes even by many government officials from the countries where NTDs are endemic. An important reason for the lack of awareness about these conditions is that the NTDs are seldom found in capital cities, where the government officials work and live. Instead, the NTDs are primarily found in poor

Table 1.4 Major attributes of the NTDs

Most prevalent among poor people
Endemic in rural areas (some poor urban areas) of low-income countries
Ancient ("the biblical diseases")
Chronic
Disabling (growth delays, blindness, or disfigurement)
Associated with high disease burden but low mortality
Stigmatizing
Poverty promoting

rural areas, particularly in regions where subsistence farming is practiced.[6] Therefore, unlike HIV/AIDS or other better-known infections, the NTDs are frequently both out of sight and out of mind. They truly are forgotten diseases afflicting forgotten people. There are exceptions, such as dengue fever and leptospirosis, which are also found in urban slums. These conditions will be addressed separately (in chapter 8), but for the most part the NTDs occur in the setting of rural poverty.

3. *The NTDs are ancient conditions.* Another interesting feature of the NTDs is their nonemerging character. By this phrase, I mean the NTDs are just the opposite of better-known *emerging infections*, such as avian influenza, SARS, Ebola, Lyme disease, West Nile virus infection, and HIV/AIDS, which have either newly appeared in the population or have rapidly increased in incidence or geographic range. Instead, the NTDs have been around seemingly forever, as they have plagued humankind for centuries. This historical link is well documented through the accounts and descriptions of some of the dramatic clinical manifestations of the NTDs, particularly leprosy, dracunculiasis, schistosomiasis, hookworm infection, and trachoma in ancient texts, including the Bible, Talmud, Vedas, writings of Hippocrates, and Egyptian medical papyri.[7] One exception to this persistent state is selected NTDs that can sometimes reappear after their earlier near elimination because of public health breakdowns resulting from civil or international conflicts. Later (in chapter 7), we will see how this situation has tragically unfolded in Angola, the Democratic Republic of the Congo, and Sudan and has resulted in a reemergence of human African trypanosomiasis and kala-azar.

4. *The NTDs are chronic conditions.* Another distinguishing feature of the NTDs is that, unlike many infectious diseases with which we are familiar, the NTDs are mostly chronic infections lasting years and sometimes even decades. In some cases, poor people can suffer from NTDs for their entire lives.[6]

5. *The NTDs cause disability and disfigurement.* Even though they are infectious diseases because they are caused by microbial or multicellular pathogens, which are transmitted either from person to person or through contact with contaminated soil or water or through exposure to arthropod vectors (e.g., mosquitoes, sandflies, assassin bugs, and copepods), the NTDs frequently do not exhibit the classic features of most infections. That is to say,

they do not typically cause acute febrile illnesses, which either resolve or kill. Instead, the NTDs mostly cause chronic conditions that lead to long-term disabilities and, in some cases, disfigurement.[6] I will highlight the specific disabling features of each of the NTDs when they are treated separately (in chapters 2 to 9), but to provide some specific examples here, the long-term effects of chronic hookworm infection and schistosomiasis in childhood produce a long-standing anemia, which is associated with physical growth retardation, impaired memory, and cognitive growth delays; in pregnant women, the anemia from hookworm infection and from schistosomiasis results in poor birth outcomes such as low neonatal birth weight and increased maternal morbidity and mortality. Onchocerciasis and trachoma cause impaired vision and blindness. Chagas' disease causes a chronic and severely disabling heart condition. LF onchocerciasis, guinea worm infection, leishmaniasis, Buruli ulcer, and leprosy cause either limb disuse or profound disfigurement (including genital deformities), which often prevent afflicted individuals from either obtaining or maintaining employment (Fig. 1.1).

6. *The NTDs have a high disease burden but low mortality.* An estimated 530,000 people die annually from the NTDs.[8] While this number of people is significant and more than twice the number estimated to have perished in the 2004 Christmas tsunami, for example, the reality is that these numbers pale in comparison to the number of annual deaths from HIV/AIDS or malaria (about 1 to 3 million deaths annually from each disease). Therefore, placing NTDs on the health radar screen of world leaders and policymakers and motivating them to tackle these conditions in a substantive way require focusing advocacy efforts on something more than simply looking at deaths as an endpoint. While it is obvious that the individuals shown in Fig. 1.1 are having their lives ruined by the long-term consequences of their NTDs, these compelling images by themselves do not provide an obvious metric that we can use to justify to the global community investments either in this group of diseases or in the people who suffer from them. Instead, we need another mechanism to convince policymakers that the "other diseases" deserve the same international attention as HIV/AIDS and malaria.

One approach to measuring the full health impact of the NTDs is to use the disability-adjusted life years, or DALYs, which consider the number of healthy life years lost from either premature death or disability. Because of the chronic, disabling, and disfiguring components of the NTDs, the DALYs ascribed to them are substantial. Shown in Table 1.5 is a ranking of HIV/AIDS, malaria, tuberculosis, and the NTDs by deaths and DALYs. One of the greatest values in DALYs is that they facilitate the comparison of one condition with another. The data illustrate that the total disability resulting from the NTDs is almost as great as the disability from HIV/AIDS and even more than the disability resulting from malaria or tuberculosis.[8]

The devastating comparison between the NTDs and the "big three" diseases, HIV/AIDS, malaria, and tuberculosis, has multiple implications for international efforts to control or eliminate infectious diseases. Today,

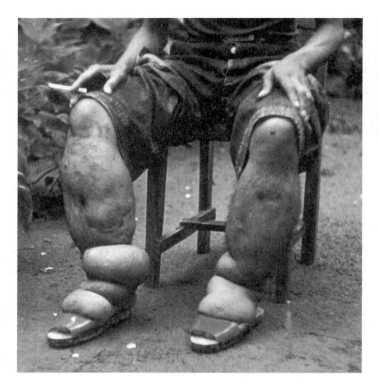

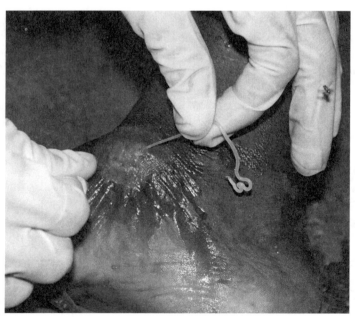

Figure 1.1 Disfiguring effects of the NTDs. (Top) Elephantiasis of the leg due to filariasis. Luzon, the Philippines (Public Health Image Library, CDC [http://phil.cdc.gov]). (Bottom) Guinea worm infection, with female worm emerging from the lower extremity (courtesy The Carter Center).

Table 1.5 Ranking of the "gang of four" by deaths and DALYs[a]

Condition	No. of DALYs annually
HIV/AIDS	84.5 million
NTDs	56.6 million
Malaria	46.5 million
Tuberculosis	34.7 million

[a]Modified from Hotez et el., 2006d.

much of the global enterprise targeting infections focuses primarily on HIV/AIDS, malaria, and tuberculosis. The DALY measurements suggest a strong rationale for considering the NTDs an important fourth leg of the chair. The rationale goes beyond merely comparing DALY estimates and pointing out the high disease burden resulting from the NTDs. Instead, an increasing body of evidence indicates not only that the NTDs exhibit geographic overlap and coendemicity with each other but also that, in addition, the NTDs are coendemic with AIDS and malaria. The geographic overlap and coendemicity between the NTDs and malaria and AIDS will be further elucidated elsewhere (chapter 10). However, to briefly mention it here, there is new evidence that the morbidities resulting from the NTDs are additive with HIV/AIDS and malaria and that, in some cases, the NTDs actually increase susceptibility to HIV/AIDS and malaria.[8] Therefore, there is an important rationale for not simply tackling the big three conditions in isolation as presently advocated by the Global Fund, PEPFAR, and PMI, but also for embracing the NTDs to take on what is really a "gang of four." This concept of integrating NTD control measures with those for malaria and HIV/AIDS will become clearer when we outline possible intervention strategies for NTD control (in chapter 10) and give the reason why we need to consider bundling treatment strategies for the NTDs together with those for HIV/AIDS and malaria (and even possibly why the Global Fund should incorporate NTD control into its programs).

7. *The NTDs are stigmatizing.* Not surprisingly, the blinding and disfiguring ravages of NTDs are stigmatizing and cause individuals to be ostracized by their families, their communities, and sometimes even health care professionals.[6] In some societies, NTDs are considered a sign of a curse or an "evil eye." The social stigma of the NTDs strikes young women particularly hard. As a result, these women are frequently abandoned by their husbands, prevented from holding or kissing their children, or unable to marry altogether. Specific examples of these stigmatizing consequences of the NTDs will be illustrated in the chapters dealing with LF, Buruli ulcer, and leishmaniasis (chapters 4, 6, and 7, respectively).

8. *The NTDs have poverty-promoting features and other socioeconomic consequences.* The health impact of the NTDs may also represent only the tip of the iceberg in terms of their adverse effects on international development. Because of their chronic and disabling features, the NTDs also produce important and serious socioeconomic consequences that keep affected

populations mired in poverty. The NTDs not only occur in the setting of poverty; they also actually promote poverty. For example, the cognitive and intellectual impairments resulting from hookworm-associated iron deficiency and anemia severely affect childhood education in terms of school performance and school attendance. Reduced school attendance leads to reduced future wage-earning capacity, possibly by as much as 43%, while chronic hookworm infection among agricultural workers has been shown to reduce worker productivity in Africa, Asia, and the Americas.[9] Similarly, LF has a huge impact on productive capacity and costs a significant percentage of India's gross national product, trachoma causes US$5.3 billion in worldwide losses annually, and leishmaniasis is responsible for 0.43% of French Guiana's social security budget.[9] We are only beginning to understand the full economic impact of the NTDs, but these nascent studies indicate that the effects are likely to be profound.

However, even a full consideration of the enormous disability, disfigurement, and economic impact does not adequately convey the total devastation wrought by the NTDs. In an interview with a Sri Lankan LF-affected patient suffering from a severe limb deformity, we can get a palpable sense of the enormous shame and stigma from the limb or genital deformities caused by her disease and how they in turn promote an inexorable slide into poverty.[10]

I got this big leg when I was engaged to be married. When they heard it was filarial, they backed out of the marriage. I was earning Rs 2,500 (US$25) a month from sewing, but when the leg got worse, the hospital doctor told me I should not pedal the machine. So I lost my income as well. When my parents died and my sister got married, only my brother and I lived in the house. My brother married and left the house, but my sister become widowed so she came to live with me and her child. She had no money to buy a bandage as instructed by the clinic. So I went to a house to cook. When they saw my leg, they asked me not to come there anymore and found fault with me for hiding such a dirty illness from them. When I get fever, I cannot walk to the hospital, so I take paracetamol for 2 days and walk to the hospital when I feel less pain.

According to the Sri Lankan health care team investigating such cases of LF, the woman in this vignette, who previously lived on earnings of approximately US$1 per day, lost even this meager income and became totally dependent on her brother-in-law.[10] An important theme in the succeeding chapters is how stigma actually contributes to the morbidity of the NTDs and creates not only a medical crisis for the affected individual but also a tragic cycle of social and economic devastation for both the individual and his family. According to the Swiss Tropical Institute's Mitchell Weiss, the stigma of the NTDs contributes to suffering, delays searching for help, promotes nonadherence to treatment, negatively impacts families and communities, and ultimately lessens support for services, control, and research.[11] Later, we will even see how, with some of the NTDs such as leishmaniasis, the stigma is particularly acute for young women, often leading to their verbal and physical abuse (in chapter 7), or how the stigma associated with Buruli ulcer is linked to beliefs about witchcraft (in chapter 6).

In summary, the health impact of the NTDs reflects their chronic and disabling features. But there are also educational and socioeconomic consequences that may even be greater. Neglect occurs at many different levels: at the community level because the NTDs arouse fear and inflict stigmas, at the national level because the NTDs occur in remote areas and are often a low priority for health ministers, and at the international level because they are not perceived as global health threats equivalent to the high-mortality big three conditions.[12] Also internationally, there has been a dearth of research and development activities concerning the NTDs; later (in chapter 11) we will see how only 0.6% of the new drugs developed over the past few decades were developed for NTDs.[12] Paul Hunt, the UN Special Rapporteur on the right to the highest attainable standard of health, points out that relief from the suffering caused by the NTDs is a fundamental human right, which unfortunately has been largely ignored.[13] Despite their global importance, we so far have no Bono equivalent to champion the plight of the 1 billion of the world's poorest people who suffer from NTDs, and the total dollars thus far committed to NTD control are presently measured in the millions, not the billions. Fortunately, this picture of neglect may yet change, in part because of a new resolve by the WHO and national ministries of health, together with several key public-private partnerships dedicated to NTD control. Further, many of the organizations involved in NTD control have begun to partner through a new alliance known as the Global Network for NTDs (discussed in chapter 10).[14] The Global Network is working to mobilize resources for the NTDs and to promote high-level advocacy from global leaders and celebrities, including former presidents Clinton and Carter, as well as Jeffrey Sachs, television star Alyssa Milano, WHO Secretary General Margaret Chan, and others. At the same time, student groups are beginning to voice their concerns about the urgency of addressing the NTDs.[15] These important, nascent efforts are about to lead to a modest revolution in global health and to make a huge impact on the world's poorest people.

Summary Points: the NTDs

- The NTDs are among the most common infections of the world's poorest people, those living on less than US$2 per day.
- Nonemerging, ancient conditions
- Chronic and disabling features
- High morbidity, low mortality
- DALYs equivalent to those for HIV/AIDS, malaria, and tuberculosis
- Coendemicity of the NTDs and with HIV/AIDS and malaria
- The "gang of four"
- Poverty-promoting features that keep populations destitute
- Associated with profound stigma
- Urgent need for stepped-up advocacy and resource mobilization

"The Unholy Trinity": the Soil-Transmitted Helminth Infections Ascariasis, Trichuriasis, and Hookworm Infection

As it was when I first saw it, so it is now, one of the most evil of infections. Not with dramatic pathology as are filariasis, or schistosomiasis, but with damage silent and insidious. Now that malaria is being pushed back, hookworm remains the great infection of mankind. In my view it outranks all other worm infections of man combined ... in its production, frequently unrealized, of human misery, debility, and inefficiency in the tropics.

NORMAN STOLL

The neglected tropical diseases (NTDs) are the most common infections of the world's poorest people, and the soil-transmitted helminth (STH) infections are the most common NTDs. The word helminth comes from the Greek ἑλμίνς, meaning "worm,"[1] and the phrase "soil-transmitted" refers to the human acquisition of these worms through contact with soil contaminated with either parasite eggs or immature larval stages. STHs are also sometimes called intestinal helminths or intestinal worms because the adult stages of the parasite live in the human gastrointestinal tract. The STHs are also nematodes, a type of parasitic worm distinguished by their elongate and cylindroidal shape.

The three most important STH infections of humans, based on their prevalence and global disease burden, are:

- *Ascaris* infection (also known as roundworm infection or ascariasis)
- *Trichuris* infection (whipworm infection or trichuriasis)
- Hookworm infection (hookworm)

Table 2.1 The "unholy trinity"

Species	Common name	Length as adult (males and females)	Major location in the GI[a] tract	No. of cases worldwide	Major disease other than impairment of child growth and development	Global distribution
Ascaris lumbricoides	Roundworm	15–35 cm (5–14 in.)	Small intestine	807 million	Intestinal obstruction	Asia, Africa, Americas
Trichuris trichiura	Whipworm	3–5 cm (1–2 in.)	Large intestine (colon)	604 million	Colitis, dysentery	Africa, Asia, Americas
N. americanus and *A. duodenale*	Hookworm	7–13 mm (0.3–0.5 in.)	Small intestine	576 million	Iron deficiency anemia	Africa, Asia, Americas

[a]GI, gastrointestinal.

Together, these helminth infections afflict over 1 billion people in developing countries.

Humans have been infected with STHs since ancient times. We know this from accurate descriptions found in Egyptian medical papyri and the writings of Hippocrates in the 5th century BCE, including reports of large *Ascaris* roundworms being expelled from infected people and of the characteristic pallor and sallow complexion found on people with hookworm.[1] In addition, STH eggs have been recovered from coprolites, mummified feces thousands of years old, found in both the Old World and New World.[1] Today, an estimated 807 million, 604 million, and 576 million people are infected with ascariasis, trichuriasis, and hookworm, respectively (Table 2.1).[2] More often than not, a single individual living in a developing country, especially a school-age child, is infected with two and sometimes all three types of STH parasites simultaneously. Practically speaking, this observation means that the intestines of hundreds of millions of children living in Africa, Asia, and the Americas harbor a menagerie of worms. Harold Brown, the late former parasitology professor at Columbia University College of Physicians and Surgeons, frequently referred to *Ascaris*, *Trichuris*, and hookworms as "the unholy trinity" to indicate that it was extremely common for a child to be infected with all three parasites simultaneously. Typically, *Ascaris* roundworms and hookworms inhabit the small intestine, while *Trichuris* whipworms inhabit the large intestine.

How can we fathom the notion of approximately 1 billion people infected with STHs? To understand this concept better, we need to travel to a developing country where STH infections are endemic, meaning that the infections are constantly present in a particular region. Figure 2.1 shows children living in a rural village in Minas Gerais State, Brazil. The families of these children are mostly subsistence farmers involved with cultivation of manioc and beans. Looking at these children, one might not think that they appear terribly ill, unless one examines them more closely. The STH-infected children living in

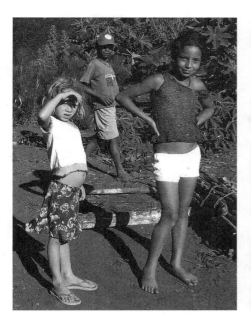
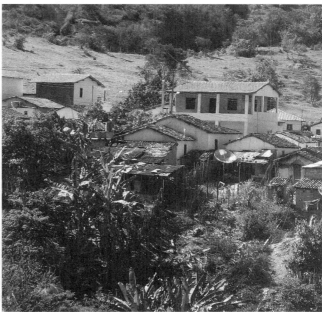

Figure 2.1 Children (left) living outside the Brazilian village of Americaninhas, Minas Gerais State (right). About 75% of people living in the area are infected with hookworm. The effects of the disease—malnutrition and anemia—are worse in children. Pictures of the children are courtesy of Brigid McCarthy of National Public Radio (© 2005 NPR).

this Brazilian village are stunted in both weight and height because they are not growing normally. Moreover, they also do poorly on tests of cognition, memory, and intelligence. There is now strong evidence that such physical and mental disabilities result from the presence of intestinal worms.[3]

The reason why we know that most of the children of Americaninhas, Minas Gerais State, Brazil, harbor intestinal worms is that we can diagnose their STH infections by examining their feces under a microscope. The adult male and female roundworms, whipworms, and hookworms mate in the intestines and produce eggs that exit the body in feces. Each type of STH produces characteristically shaped eggs that are easy to identify through microscopy. If we now do this test for all children in this particular rural Brazilian village, we get a result that is shown in Fig. 2.2, in which more than 70% of the children between the ages of 5 and 11 are infected with *Ascaris* worms and hookworms. It turns out that we can repeat this study in almost any rural Brazilian village or indeed almost any rural village in the tropical regions of the Americas, including Central America, and probably obtain a similar result or find that just as many children are also infected with *Trichuris* whipworms. Indeed, if we were to conduct fecal examinations in most of the rural villages in sub-Saharan Africa, on the Indian subcontinent, or in Southeast Asia, really wherever people live in poverty and depend on subsistence agriculture and where the soil and

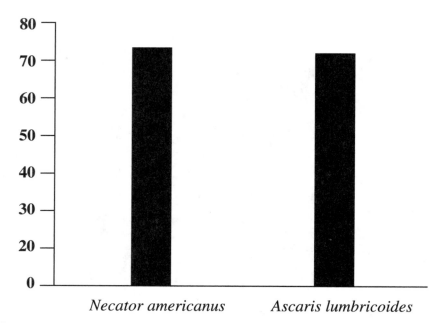

Figure 2.2 Prevalence of STH infections among school-age children in Americaninhas, Brazil (data courtesy of Jeff Bethony and David Diemert, Human Hookworm Vaccine Initiative; modified from graph prepared by Sophia Raff).

climate are suitable for survival of the parasite eggs and immature larval stages (typically the warm and moist soil of the tropics), we would find a similar paradigm of extraordinarily high rates of STH infections. Such observations suggest how it can be that hundreds of millions of people harbor the unholy trinity in their bellies.

Beginning in the late 1980s, parasitologists of the Chinese Academy of Preventive Medicine, now known as the Chinese Center for Disease Control and Prevention, conducted a four-year study of intestinal parasites on an almost unimaginable scale by performing fecal examinations on 1,477,742 individuals in every province of China. The results were impressive and demonstrated that, if we extrapolate for the entire Chinese population, approximately 531 million cases of ascariasis, 212 million cases of trichuriasis, and 194 million cases of hookworm infection had occurred in that country.[4] In collaboration with the Institute of Parasitic Diseases in Shanghai, I began working in China shortly after the completion of this nationwide survey of parasites. What particularly impressed me was the very tight link between high endemicity of STH infections in rural China and the level of economic underdevelopment.[5] Wherever rural poverty was extreme and the villagers were engaged in subsistence agriculture, and provided that there were suitable moisture and warmth, it was almost guaranteed that high levels of hookworm and other STH infections were present. Conversely, in areas of rapid economic gains, the STH disappeared. For instance, during the late 1990s when I visited a village in Jiangsu Province, not too far from Shanghai, there had been a steep decline in the prevalence of hookworm from just a decade previously.[6] The decline coincided with the building of new factories so that fewer villagers were engaged in agricultural activities. Moreover, there was even a new Kentucky Fried Chicken franchise, as well as a pirated version with the same red and white logos—called KCF instead of KFC! Hookworm occurs only in the setting of poverty, and, in a sense, the factory, KFC, and KCF represent indicators of economic development.

As shown in Fig. 2.3, the relationship between STH prevalence and poverty is extremely tight,[7] and I believe that it is feasible to develop a "worm index" of economic development as a poverty indicator. However, a clear understanding of the specific mechanisms underlying the link between a high prevalence of STH infections and poverty is still somewhat elusive. At least three possible factors linking poverty to STH infections have been identified so far, including (i) inadequate sanitation, because survival of the environmental stages of STH parasites depends on the deposition of human feces on soil; (ii) poor housing construction, because dirt floors allow propagation of STHs in households, while cement floors prevent parasite transmission; and (iii) inadequate access to essential medicines, because better-off families can

Figure 2.3 The relationship between prevalence of hookworm and poverty. The socioeconomic status of 94 countries was assessed according to a number of commonly used indicators, with poverty measures divided into quartiles including the poorest (first quartile), very poor (second quartile), poor (third quartile), and least poor (fourth quartile). Original comes from de Silva et al., 2003. Figure was later modified for Hotez et al., 2005.

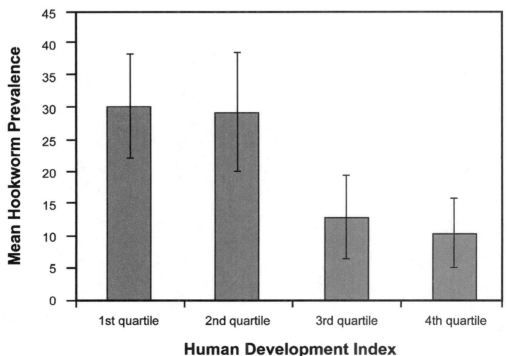

afford deworming drugs.[8] Urbanization is also a potent factor in reducing the prevalence of STH infections. In eastern China, for example, rapid economic growth has brought with it a significant decline in prevalence, while in the poor and largely rural southern and southwestern provinces of China, such as Hainan, Sichuan, Yunnan, and Guangxi, hookworm and other STH infections remain highly endemic.[5,8]

In addition to their enormous global prevalence and their intimate link with rural poverty, another important feature of the STH infections is their predilection for affecting children more than adults. For reasons that are not well understood, children between the ages of 4 and 15 on average harbor larger numbers of STHs than do any other group; i.e., children are wormier than adults. This propensity is particularly true for *Ascaris* roundworms and *Trichuris* whipworms, less so for hookworms. For example, shown in Fig. 2.4 is a little girl from Paraguay who simultaneously is emaciated and has a distended abdomen. It is sometimes possible to gently palpate the abdomens of children like her and feel the presence of worms in their intestines. Figure 2.4 also shows

Figure 2.4 (Left) Little girl from Paraguay with severe *Ascaris* worm infection. Picture is courtesy of Nora Labiano and reproduced from Despommier et al., 2006. (Right) Worms expelled after anthelmintic treatment.

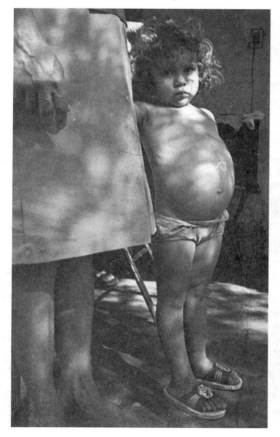 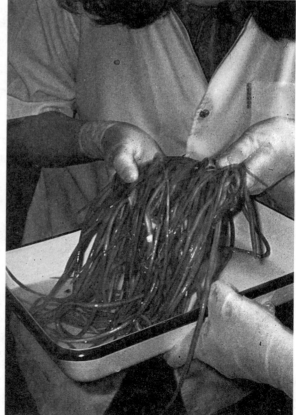

the *Ascaris* roundworms that she expelled after treatment with an anthelmintic drug (a process often referred to as deworming). It is easy to grasp how this girl could get into medical trouble if the roundworms were allowed to remain and obstruct the intestine or in some cases migrate from the intestine and into the liver or pancreas. When children harbor large numbers of whipworms in their colon, the resulting chronic inflammation can cause rectal prolapse, i.e., a telescoping of the rectum that protrudes from the anus.

Although such clinical pictures are dramatic, they actually represent only a small portion of the global pediatric pathology caused by STHs. Far more important is the observation that in hundreds of millions of children the STHs stunt physical growth, physical fitness, and development. These processes probably operate at least partly through parasite-induced malnutrition, as all three major STHs can live in the intestines of children for years, where they can rob children of essential nutrients. For example, *Ascaris* roundworm infections most likely retard growth by impairing the digestion of protein, causing the malabsorption of fat, lactose, and vitamin A, as well as reducing appetite; *Trichuris* whipworm infections also result in reduced appetite, as well as in protein losses; and hookworms impair growth by causing blood loss that leads to profound protein and iron losses and ultimately to anemia.[9] Through these mechanisms, it is possible that STHs represent the world's leading cause of growth retardation and stunting!

Moreover, the unholy trinity also adversely affects the neuropsychiatric activities of children, in turn damaging school performance and reducing school attendance.[10,11] The mechanisms by which school performance is impaired are not well established, but a number of clinical studies have shown that STHs can adversely affect cognition and memory and in some cases possibly lower intelligence.[11] Therefore, chronic infections with STHs destroy the lives of children not by shortening their lives but instead by impairing their physical growth, mental development, and ability to learn in school. Each of the NTDs not only occurs in the setting of poverty but also promotes poverty. In the case of STH infections, roundworms, whipworms, and hookworms promote poverty primarily through their impact on overall child development. Presumably, these processes account for the observation that chronic infection with hookworm during childhood is associated with a 43% reduction in future wage-earning capacity (similar studies for ascariasis and trichuriasis are not yet available).[12] Therefore, STH infections have a huge impact not only on health but also on education, and like other NTDs they are economic threats.

As suggested by the opening quotation from the late Norman Stoll, hookworm is probably the most significant STH. Hookworms are 1-cm-long parasites that live in the small intestine, where they suck blood from the small blood vessels lining the gut mucosa and submucosa. Almost 600 million people, approximately one-fourth of the world's poorest people, are infected with hookworm. The greatest concentration of cases occurs in rural areas of sub-Saharan Africa (198 million cases), East Asia and the Pacific region (149 million cases), the Indian subcontinent (130 million cases), and tropical regions of the Americas (50 million cases), especially Brazil and Central America (Color

Plate 2).[2,13] Infection rates are often particularly high in coastal areas, an observation that most likely reflects the unique requirements of the soil-dwelling environmental stages of these parasites.

Nearly as striking as the high prevalence of hookworm in developing countries is the almost complete absence of hookworm in developed countries, including the United States. However, up until the 1930s, hookworm infection (as well as many other NTDs, such as malaria and typhoid fever) was endemic in the southern United States.[14] Shown in Color Plate 3 is a map of the distribution of hookworm in the American South during the first decades of the 20th century, when high rates of hookworm infection occurred along the Gulf Coast and the Atlantic seaboard (the basis for the high rates of hookworm in coastal areas will become clearer when we discuss the hookworm life cycle). In some regions where more than 50% of the children were infected, it was shown that hookworm was a major reason why children were malnourished, why their growth was stunted, and why they did poorly in school and were prevented from reaching their full economic potential.[12,14]

After Charles Wardell Stiles and Bailey K. Ashford identified *Necator americanus* as the predominant hookworm in the United States, it became known as the "germ of laziness" or the "vampire of the South."[1,14] It is believed that hookworm was introduced into the United States when *N. americanus* was imported by infected slaves from sub-Saharan Africa during the 17th, 18th, and 19th centuries.[1,14] Up until the 1950s, hookworm was also common in Japan and South Korea. In each of these now developed countries, reductions in the prevalence of tropical infections occurred primarily because of overall reductions in poverty and a shift to a more urbanized economy. In her book *Malaria, Poverty, Race, and Public Health in the United States*, the medical historian Margaret Humphreys argues that the Agricultural Adjustment Act and other New Deal legislation, which Congress passed in 1933, promoted rural depopulation by providing investment capital for the purchase of machinery, which took agricultural workers out of cotton and tobacco production.[15] Such legislation caused landlords to tear down rural shacks and forced former dwellers to move either north or into southern cities.[15] There is a common misconception that, during the first two decades of the 20th century, the Rockefeller Foundation and its forerunner, the Rockefeller Sanitary Commission, eradicated hookworm in the American South and later in parts of Asia and South America through a combination of aggressive sanitation and the widespread distribution of shoes. For reasons that we will see below, it turns out that shoes are not an effective hookworm prevention measure, while sanitation in the absence of parallel economic development has a remarkably small impact on the transmission of STH infections.[16] Instead, rural depopulation in the United States during the 1930s and in Japan and Korea in the years following World War II was the major element leading to control of STH infections. Control was further hastened through widespread deworming by using first-generation anthelmintic drugs. Similar changes in human ecology probably account for the reductions observed in eastern China over the last 2 decades. Therefore, urbanization and economic development represent two of the most powerful forces responsible for the control of hookworm infection and other NTDs. Far more than the Sanitary Commission, the major health legacy of John Rockefeller was his foresight in establishing The Rockefeller University as a biomedical research powerhouse and in endowing the first generation of public health schools in the United States, beginning with the flagship school at Johns Hopkins University.

Humans become infected with hookworm through contact with infective larvae that live in the soil.[17] The major cause of human hookworm infection is the nematode parasite *N. americanus*, although a second but less common species, *Ancylostoma duodenale*, also causes hookworm infection. The life cycle of *N. americanus* is shown in Fig. 2.5. Soil-dwelling infective hookworm larvae exhibit the ability to directly penetrate human skin. The larvae are less than 1 mm long (Color Plate 4) and therefore largely invisible to people working in the fields or children playing on the ground. Larvae enter through any exposed skin, including the hands, the arms, the buttocks, the legs, and, yes,

Figure 2.5 Life cycle of the hookworm *N. americanus* (from Hotez et al., 2005).

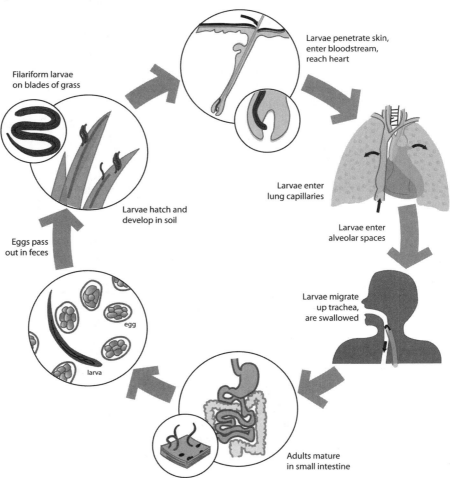

Filariform larvae on blades of grass

Larvae penetrate skin, enter bloodstream, reach heart

Larvae enter lung capillaries

Larvae hatch and develop in soil

Eggs pass out in feces

Larvae enter alveolar spaces

Larvae migrate up trachea, are swallowed

egg

larva

Adults mature in small intestine

sometimes even the feet. The ability of *N. americanus* larvae to penetrate all aspects of the skin explains why shoes have minimal if any impact on reducing the hookworm prevalence in affected communities. The higher rates of hookworm infection in coastal areas reflect the sandy soils present in this region. Hookworm larvae can migrate through sandy soils better than through soils with a high clay content.[18]

It is common for people exposed repeatedly to hookworm larvae in the soil to acquire a pruritic (itchy) inflammatory condition of the skin known as ground itch or dew itch. The larvae then follow a 5- to 8-week migratory path through the body tissues, which includes an obligatory migration through the lungs that results in a cough (in contrast, when *Ascaris* larvae migrate through the lungs, they cause wheezing and other allergic symptoms that resemble asthma). Eventually, the infective hookworm larvae pass up the respiratory tree, crawl over the epiglottis, and are swallowed before they enter the intestine and develop into adult hookworms. Each adult hookworm has the ability to fasten deeply to the inner lining of the intestine and extract blood. The parasite lyses red blood cells and digests the hemoglobin component.[19] While feeding, the adult male and female hookworms mate and the female hookworm sheds thousands of eggs daily, which exit the body via the feces. In poor rural environments lacking adequate sanitation, either promiscuous defecation occurs or, in some societies, human feces are used to fertilize crops (in such cases, they are sometimes referred to as night soil). When feces are deposited on soil with adequate warmth and moisture, the eggs hatch and give rise to immature larvae that molt to become infective larvae.

People infected with hookworms become sick because of intestinal blood loss. The presence of as few as 25 *N. americanus* hookworms in the intestine is sufficient to cause about 1 ml of blood loss per day.[20] This amount of blood contains approximately 0.5 mg of iron, representing roughly a typical child's daily iron requirement. Therefore, hookworms essentially rob growing children of their daily iron and, as a result, cause iron deficiency anemia.[20] Higher hookworm loads cause even more blood loss and more profound anemia. Therefore, the disease resulting from chronic hookworm infection (sometimes referred to as hookworm disease) is long-standing iron deficiency anemia, which in children is responsible for growth retardation and intellectual and cognitive impairments. Because children tend to have low iron reserves from the outset, they are particularly vulnerable to hookworm-associated blood loss. Blood is also rich in protein, so that chronic blood loss can result in profound protein malnutrition, which is associated with edema of the face and limbs (Fig. 2.6). Many such children acquire a yellowish or sallow complexion; in several cultures, hookworm is known as the "yellow disease" or the "yellow puffy disease" (in Chinese, *huang zhong bing*, and in Brazilian Portuguese, *amarelao*). In antiquity, there are numerous references to the yellow disease, and there is an older term in the English medical literature, chlorosis, that refers to this condition.[17] Another unusual feature of chronic hookworm infection is pica, an appetite for consuming clay and other bulky substances. Referring to hookworm, Hippocrates described a syndrome in which "the skin is yellow, the intestine disturbed, and the person has an appetite for eating clay," and there

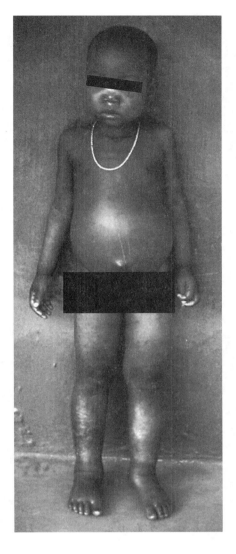

Figure 2.6 Severe hookworm disease. The child is both pale and edematous, thus reflecting severe loss of both iron and protein (Public Health Image Library, CDC [http://phil.cdc.gov.]).

are numerous references to clay eating in early Southern culture.[1] It has been suggested that eating clay represents an effort to replace iron stores because of its high iron content.[1]

Hookworm is also an important health threat during pregnancy, and an estimated 44 million pregnant women worldwide suffer from hookworm infection. Pregnant women typically have low iron reserves and are often iron deficient to begin with. There is a strong link between the added iron losses and anemia that result from hookworm and adverse maternal-fetal outcomes such as neonatal prematurity, low birth weight, and increased maternal mortality.[20,21] Among agricultural laborers, chronic hookworm iron deficiency results in impaired worker productivity and productive capacity (Fig. 2.7). In the early part of the 20th century, the Brazilian writer Monteiro Lobato created the now famous character of Jeca Tatu, a laborer who is always lazy and lacking in energy until he is cured of his hookworm infection and then goes on to champion social causes (Fig. 2.7). The chronic disabilities associated with impaired child development, poor pregnancy outcome, and worker productivity account for the observation that hookworm costs more healthy life years lost through disability (DALYs) annually than any other parasitic worm infection.[22]

Given that shoes do not protect against hookworm infection, what might be our options for controlling or preventing hookworm in developing countries? The sanitary disposal of human feces by increased use of latrines could under some circumstances dramatically reduce the prevalence of hookworm and other STH infections. However, the best evidence to date is that, unless it is accompanied by substantial poverty reduction measures and urbanization, the isolated use of latrines has minimal, if any, impact on the transmission of hookworm or other STH infections.[16] Presently, the most effective approach to the control of STH infections is through deworming of large populations through mass drug administration of a specific anthelmintic with the ability

Figure 2.7 (Left) A Brazilian worker with *amarelao*, chronic hookworm infection (from Klintowitz, 1989). (Right) Jeca Tatu.

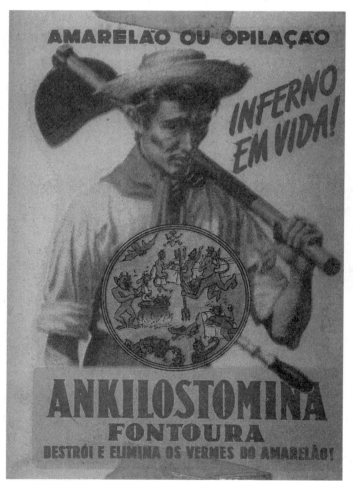
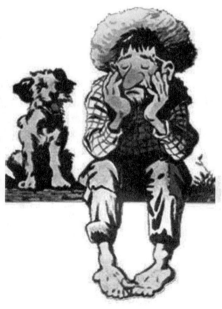

to expel all three major parasite species. This approach is the first example that we will describe in which mass drug administration (frequently abbreviated as MDA) is used for the large-scale control or elimination of an NTD.

For the STHs, anthelmintic drugs belonging to the benzimidazole class (sometimes referred to as benzimidazole anthelmintics or BZAs) are primarily used in a single dose for purposes of mass deworming. The two major available BZAs are albendazole and mebendazole. Both drugs are available as low-cost generic products, and in some cases BZA donations are being organized through two programs housed at the Task Force for Child Development and Survival in Atlanta, including a Johnson & Johnson program for mebendazole donations and a GlaxoSmithKline program for albendazole (although in the case of the GlaxoSmithKline program, albendazole is primarily being donated for another purpose, namely, for the control of lymphatic filariasis). Because school-age children are particularly at risk for heavy STH infections with large numbers of worms, this group is the major one targeted for global deworming efforts. Frequent and periodic deworming of school-age children with BZAs has been shown to result in a number of pediatric health and nutritional benefits, including improvements in appetite, physical fitness, and physical growth, as well as improved iron status and reductions in anemia.[11,23] Deworming also produces neuropsychiatric progress, including positive intellectual and cognitive effects, such as improvements to short-term and long-term memory, problem solving, language skills, and cognition.[11,23] Therefore, BZA deworming produces educational benefits as well as health benefits, including a reduction in school absenteeism.[10,11,23]

Every May, the world's ministers of health meet at the annual World Health Assembly, held at WHO headquarters in Geneva, Switzerland. At the 54th World Health Assembly in 2001, a resolution was adopted (Resolution 54.19) that urged member nations to attain a minimum target of regular deworming of at least 75% and up to 100% of all at-risk school-age children (http://www.who.int/wormcontrol). Since then, there has been heightened advocacy by the WHO and other international agencies for the administration of BZAs, typically a single dose of either albendazole or mebendazole, on a large scale. Increasingly, annual deworming is being practiced in schools because of the cost-effectiveness and efficiencies of having teachers rather than health care practitioners administer anthelmintic drugs.[24] This approach includes using schoolteachers who are specially trained to deliver the deworming tablets alongside health education messaging.[23] In many African countries, deworming is linked with school feeding programs sponsored by the World Food Programme (http://www.wfp.org) through the FRESH Partnership (Focusing Resources on Effective School Health), an interagency initiative of the World Bank, UNICEF, UNESCO, and WHO (http://www.freshschools.org).[23] Such interventions can be achieved at extremely low cost. For example, in Ghana and Tanzania, hundreds of thousands of children have been treated for as little as US$0.03 and US$0.04 per capita.[23,24] One of the reasons why the costs of school-based deworming are so low is that the excellent safety profile of a single dose of a BZA allows children to be treated regardless of whether they are infected with STHs. Instead, once it is established that the overall community prevalence of STH infections exceeds 50%, it no longer becomes necessary to conduct fecal examinations on each child. Authorities can then blanket the school with a single dose of either mebendazole or albendazole. This practice eliminates the high cost of bringing trained microscopists and laboratory equipment to the school. I believe that the advocacy efforts of two individuals, namely, Lorenzo Savioli at WHO and Don Bundy, now at the World Bank, were especially instrumental in promoting global deworming and advancing the agenda leading to Resolution 54.19.[25]

To date, more than 10 million children in more than 30 countries have been treated in low-cost deworming and school feeding programs.[23] However, while this number is impressive, it is still far short of the estimated hundreds of millions of children who would need to be treated annually in order to meet the targets specified by Resolution 54.19.[26] Moreover, many school-age children do not attend school in developing countries. Therefore, as an alternative or complementary approach to school-based interventions, many children are being targeted worldwide through community-based interventions, which include child health days. In such programs, deworming is linked to vitamin A distribution as well as to some immunizations, such as measles vaccinations.[23] Child health days and other community-based interventions are particularly suitable in regions of STH infection endemicity where preschool children, i.e., children under the age of five, also suffer from moderate and heavy infections. By some estimates, almost 200 million children have received vitamin A in more than 50 countries,[23] so that this mechanism provides an added opportunity to scale up deworming. Also, as pointed out earlier, in some developing countries, pregnant women are at high risk for hookworm infection, and the WHO and other international agencies have therefore expanded their recommended targets to include this group in areas of high transmission.

Although for most school-based and community-based interventions a single dose of either mebendazole or albendazole is provided on an annual basis, in areas of intense transmission deworming may need to be conducted more frequently. This need arises because, in such areas, STH reinfection can occur over a period of just a few months, so that sometimes two or three dewormings must take place in a single year. Presently, the WHO recommends two or three deworming treatments annually in areas of high prevalence (typically greater than 70% prevalence) or high intensity (where more than 10% of the population have moderate or heavy infections).

When frequent and periodic dewormings are required in order to control STH infections for large populations, there are concerns that STH parasites, like any other infectious agent, could over time become resistant to either mebendazole or albendazole. Indeed, BZA resistance is now widespread among intestinal helminth parasites of sheep and cattle in Australia, New Zealand, South America, South Africa, and elsewhere in the Southern Hemisphere.[27] The mechanisms by which BZA resistance occur will be discussed later (in chapter 11). Today, the high rate of drug failures for single-dose mebendazole and high rates of STH infection in areas of high transmission, coupled with emerging evidence of BZA resistance in human nematodes, have led to international calls for increased monitoring and for the development of new-generation STH drugs. Given the enormous health and educational benefits of deworming, I believe that we should try to do everything possible to scale up the use of BZAs in developing countries. At the same time, however, we must try to develop backup control tools. Unfortunately, the absence of a commercial market for such drugs has hampered a substantive research and development effort on this front. As an alternative or complementary approach to STH control, there has been a concerted effort to develop a recombinant anthelmintic vaccine, which would prevent reinfection following deworming.[28] Later (in chapter 11), I will discuss the efforts of our nonprofit product development partnership, the Human Hookworm Vaccine Initiative (HHVI), to develop a new hookworm vaccine as an important antipoverty measure.

Summary Points: the STHs

- STH infections are caused by intestinal worms, with *Ascaris* roundworms, *Trichuris* whipworms, and hookworms being the most common.
- Ascariasis, trichuriasis, and hookworm infection are the world's most common NTDs.
- STH infections are highly prevalent in sub-Saharan Africa, Asia, and the Americas, especially in areas where rural poverty overlaps with tropical environments and adequate rainfall.
- Children typically exhibit heavier STH infections with higher worm burdens than do adults.
- The STHs live for years in the gastrointestinal tract.
- In children, chronic STH infections impair physical growth and development as well as cognition, memory, and school performance. Therefore, STHs produce educational deficits as well as ill health. These poverty-promoting features probably result from parasite-induced malnutrition.
- Hookworms cause malnutrition and disease when sufficiently large numbers of the parasites cause intestinal blood loss, leading to iron deficiency anemia. Hookworm disease and anemia are particularly common in children and pregnant women. The DALYs lost to hookworm infection rank the highest for any worm infection.
- Large numbers of *Ascaris* worms in the small intestine can result in acute intestinal obstruction, while large numbers of *Trichuris* worms in the large intestine can produce inflammation leading to colitis or rectal prolapse.
- Global control of STH infections presently focuses on morbidity reductions through frequent and periodic deworming with BZAs. School-based deworming is being frequently emphasized in order to target at-risk children.
- There are both theoretical and actual concerns about BZA drug resistance; a human hookworm vaccine is under development.

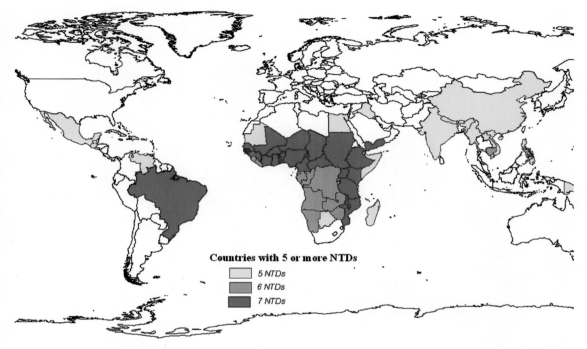

Color Plate 1 (chapter 1) Developing countries with five or more NTDs. Of the 56 nations with five or more coendemic NTDs, 40 are found in Africa, nine in Asia, five in the Americas, and two in the Middle East (map prepared by Sophia Raff).

Color Plate 2 (chapter 2) Global distribution of human hookworm infection. (From Hotez et al., 2005.)

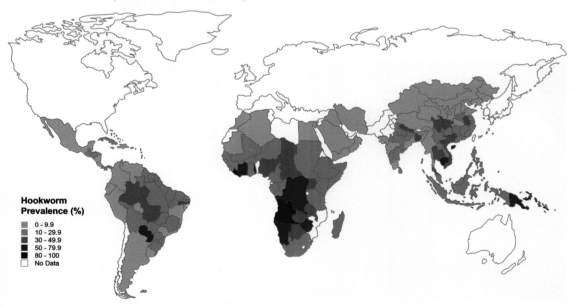

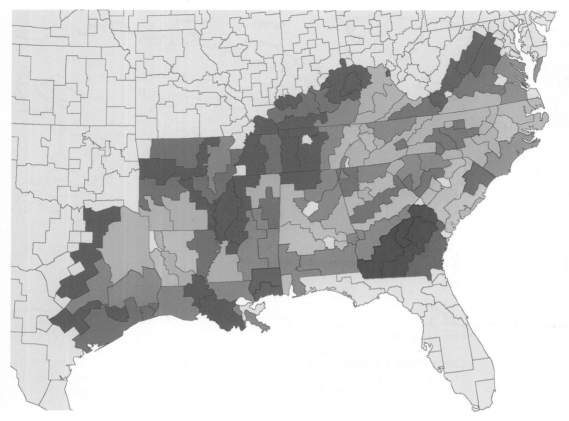

Color Plate 3 (chapter 2) Distribution of human hookworm infection in the American South at the turn of the 20th century. The map displays the rates of hookworm infection among children by county groups. Red areas indicate the highest infection rates followed by orange, yellow, and green. Data from Bleakley, 2006.

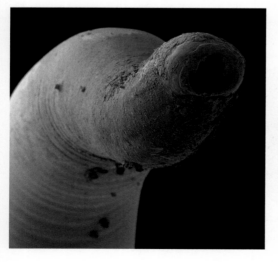

Color Plate 4 (chapter 2) Picture of an adult hookworm (courtesy of David Sharf [http://www.electronmicro.com]).

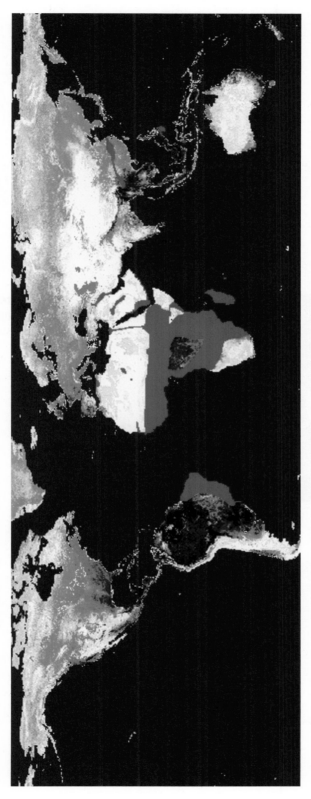

Color Plate 5 (chapter 3) The global distribution of schistosomiasis (in red) (http:// geo.arc.nasa.gov/sge/health/sensor/diseases/images/schisto.gif).

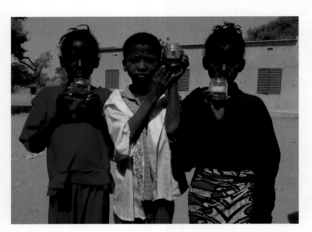

Color Plate 6 (chapter 3) Children in Niger with hematuria (photo courtesy of Juerg Utzinger, Swiss Tropical Institute).

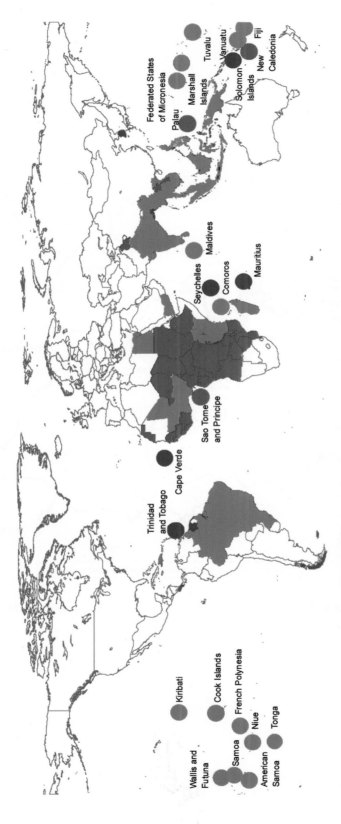

Color Plate 7 (chapter 4) Geographic distribution of LF (see http://www.filariasis. org/resources/countries_map_list.htm). Green indicates countries of endemicity in which MDA is implemented; blue indicates countries unlikely to require MDA; red indicates countries and territories where LF is endemic. (Source: ©2008, World Health Organization.)

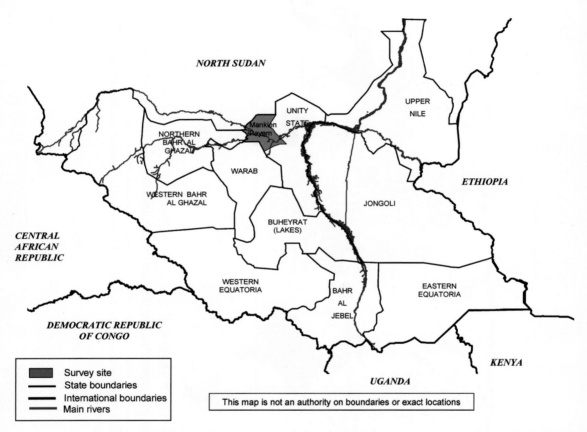

NORTH SUDAN

UNITY STATE

Mankien Payam

NORTHERN BAHR AL GHAZAL

UPPER NILE

WARAB

WESTERN BAHR AL GHAZAL

ETHIOPIA

JONGOLI

BUHEYRAT (LAKES)

CENTRAL AFRICAN REPUBLIC

WESTERN EQUATORIA

BAHR AL JEBEL

EASTERN EQUATORIA

DEMOCRATIC REPUBLIC OF CONGO

KENYA

UGANDA

Survey site
State boundaries
International boundaries
Main rivers

This map is not an authority on boundaries or exact locations

Color Plate 8 (chapter 5) Map of Southern Sudan showing the Mankien study site.

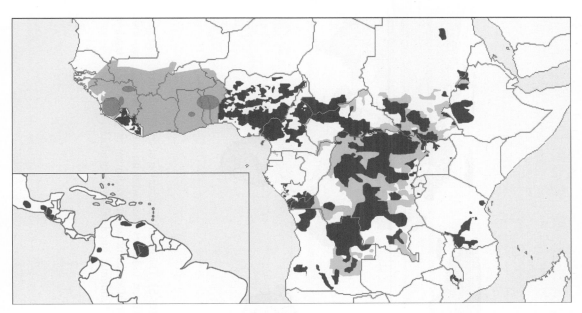

Color Plate 9 (chapter 5) Distribution of onchocerciasis showing current status of global control efforts. Red areas represent areas under ivermectin coverage, yellow areas represent areas requiring further surveillance information, green areas are those covered previously by the OCP in West Africa, and pink areas indicate special intervention zones, i.e., previous OCP areas still receiving ivermectin and some vector control. From Basanez et al., 2006.

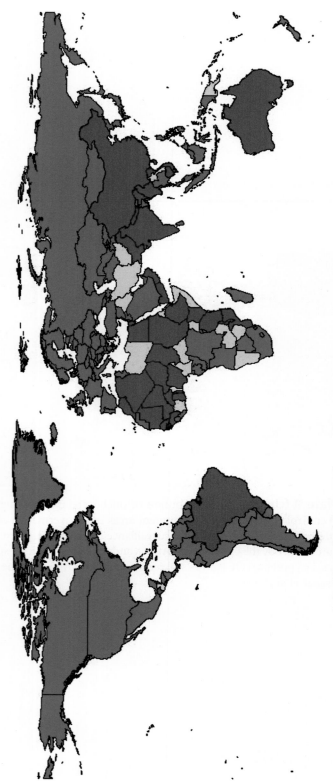

Color Plate 10 (chapter 5) The global distribution of trachoma (http://gamapserver. who.int/mapLibrary). Green indicates areas with no active trachoma; red indicates areas with data-confirmed endemic active trachoma; in yellow areas, trachoma is believed to be active and endemic, but data are not available.

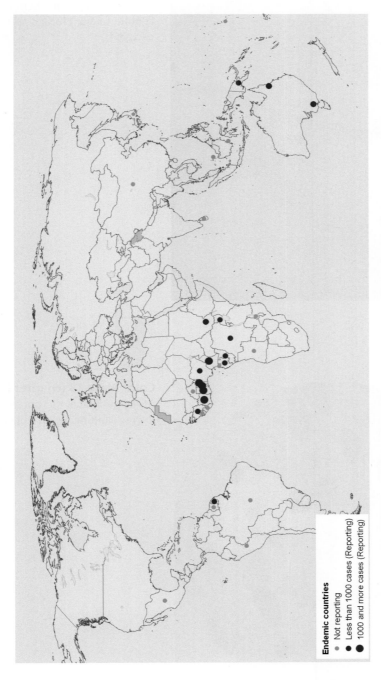

Color Plate 11 (chapter 6) Geographic distribution of Buruli ulcer. Original data source is the WHO/Global Buruli Ulcer Initiative (http://www.who.int).

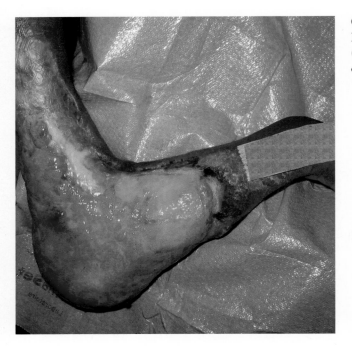

Color Plate 12 (chapter 6) Case of Buruli ulcer from Benin, West Africa (Public Image Library, CDC [http://phil.cdc.gov]).

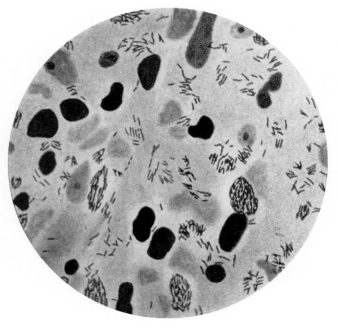

Color Plate 13 (chapter 6) Drawing of *M. leprae* under the microscope and following staining. From Rinaldi, 2005.

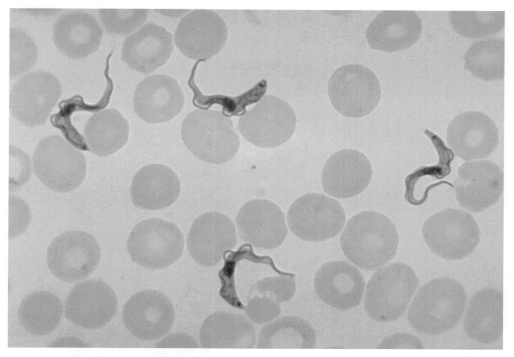

Color Plate 14 (chapter 7) Photomicrograph of stained trypanosomes in the bloodstream (Public Health Image Library, CDC [http://phil.cdc.gov]).

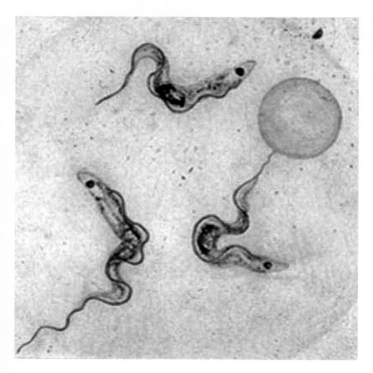

Color Plate 15 (chapter 7) Reproduction of J. E. Dutton's original watercolor drawing of *T. b. gambiense* from the blood of an infected patient. Image is from the archives of the University of Liverpool (courtesy of David H. Molyneux).

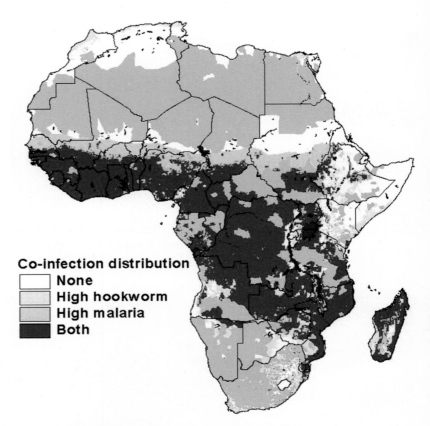

Color Plate 16 (chapter 10) Geographic overlap of moderate to high hookworm infection prevalence (>20% prevalence of infection among school-age children) and transmission of falciparum malaria (based on a map of climatic suitability for malaria transmission adjusted for urbanization). From Brooker et al., 2004.

chapter 3

Schistosomiasis (Snail Fever)

Welcome the sunrise, come under the stars, work from dusk to daybreak
Our strength is boundless, our enthusiasm is redder than fire ...
Be the river like a sea, drained clean it shall be ...
Empty the rivers to wipe out the snails, resolutely to fight the big-belly disease.

WEI WEN-PO, 1958

Schistosomiasis is a waterborne parasitic worm infection affecting 207 million people in developing countries.[1] Approximately 97% of the cases occur in the poorest regions of Africa. An additional 1 to 2 million cases each also occur in the Americas (primarily in Brazil) as well as in the Middle East (primarily in Yemen), and there are approximately 1 million cases of Asian schistosomiasis in China, the Philippines, and Southeast Asia.[1] Unlike the soil-transmitted helminths, which are nematodes, the schistosomes are a type of flatworm, also known as a trematode or fluke. As adult worms, schistosomes live in the bloodstream (and are known also as blood flukes), where they release eggs armed with a spine that produces serious disease in either the urinary tract or in the intestine and liver, depending on the particular species of parasite. Humans acquire schistosomiasis by direct contact with the larval stages (known as cercariae) that swim in freshwater. Prior to becoming cercariae, the immature developing and reproducing forms of these parasites spend a part of their life history living in various species of aquatic snails.

Few other infectious diseases have influenced history more than schistosomiasis has. Joshua's curse and the abandonment of Jericho have been attributed to the disease.[2] Schistosomiasis was well known to the ancient Egyptians, and it was a major scourge of Napoleon's army during its disastrous campaign in Egypt between 1798 and 1801.[2] However, some of the most dramatic examples of the schistosome's historical impact draw from postrevolutionary China during the second half of the 20th century. Shortly after the Chinese revolution in 1949, Mao Zedong (Mao Tse-tung) began planning a massive amphibious assault to bring Taiwan (then known as Formosa) under Communist control. While undergoing rigorous water training around the eastern tributaries of the Yangtze River, tens of thousands of People's Liberation Army (PLA) troops were exposed to the infectious cercariae of *Schistosoma japonicum*, the parasitic larvae that live in the water and are shed by snails living in the wet mud along the riverbanks. Within weeks, tens of thousands of soldiers experienced the early acute phase of schistosomiasis, a condition known as Katayama syndrome, which can last for weeks and is characterized by fever, extreme fatigue, muscle pains, and coughing.[3] As a result, the amphibious attack was delayed just long enough for the U.S. Seventh Fleet to enter the Strait of Formosa and abort a Communist takeover. These events were described in a 1959 *Harper's Magazine* article titled "The Blood Fluke That Saved Formosa."[4]

Undoubtedly, the derailment of the PLA by a blood fluke transmitted by a snail made a deep impression on the Chinese Communist Party leadership. Beginning in 1955 on the order of Chairman Mao, a special nine-man committee on schistosomiasis was established and a seven-year plan for the eradication of the disease was launched.[5] In 1958, beginning with the Great Leap Forward, millions of peasants were mobilized to the Yangtze River valley, where they drained the marshes and buried the "devil snails" under dirt or, in some cases, removed the snails individually with sticks.[6] The quotation at the opening of this chapter is from a 1958 paper written by Wei Wen-po (the second-in-command of the nine-man committee) that appeared in the *Chinese Medical Journal* under the title "The People's Boundless Energy during the Current Leap Forward."[7] Later, chemical agents to kill the snails were applied. Such low-technology interventions directed at snail control had a major important impact and helped to reduce the overall prevalence of schistosomiasis from over 12 million or more cases before the revolution to approximately 1.6 million cases by the mid-1980s.[6] Mao himself wrote a poem about these successes entitled "Farewell to the God of Plague." Today, there is new concern that the completion of the Three Gorges Dam across the Yangtze River might help to establish new ecological niches for snails to thrive and reproduce, thereby causing a rebound in the number of cases of schistosomiasis, just as other dam projects on the Nile at Aswan and the Senegal and Volta rivers in sub-Saharan Africa have caused massive increases in snail populations and reemergence of the disease.[8]

In Egypt and elsewhere in East Africa, schistosomiasis has had an equally profound historical impact. Schistosome eggs have even been recovered from Egyptian mummies dating from the 20th dynasty, around 1000 BCE.[2] During the first half of the 20th century, more than half of the populations in some rural villages of the Nile Delta were infected with either *Schistosoma haematobium* or *Schistosoma mansoni*. Both forms of schistosomiasis were considered the scourge of the *fellaheen*, Egypt's peasant agricultural laborers.[9] It was said that hematuria, the bloody urine that results from *S. haematobium* infection, was so common among Egyptian children and adolescent boys that it was considered a form of male menstruation.[9] The initial efforts to control schistosomiasis in Egypt and in neighboring Sudan (where the Gezira Scheme, one of the world's largest irrigation projects, is located near the confluence of the Blue Nile and White Nile) were organized by the British, initially through multiple injections of toxic antimony compounds to cure the disease in humans and subsequently through widespread use of molluscicides, snail-destroying chemical agents distributed in the environment.[10] During the 1960s, Bayluscide (known generically as niclosamide), a molluscicide developed by Bayer, was widely used but later largely abandoned because of price increases combined with a realization that it caused significant damage to fish and other wildlife. Subsequently, during the 1970s, newly discovered drugs, such as ambilhar and hycanthone, were used in large-scale treatment of schistosomiasis, but they too fell into disuse because of their toxicity and some unexplained deaths.[10] Finally, during the 1990s, widespread use of the anthelmintic drug praziquantel in a 14-year-long mass drug administration campaign (supported in part by the World Bank and the U.S. Agency for International Development) reduced the overall prevalence of schistosomiasis in Egypt to less than 10% of the population.[10,11] In China, a 10-year World Bank initiative also supporting mass drug administration of praziquantel has resulted in similar dramatic reductions of schistosomiasis in the Yangtze River valley.[10]

Despite the successes in China and Egypt, today schistosomiasis still rivals hookworm infection as the most important helminth infection of humans. Urinary schistosomiasis caused by *S. haematobium* is responsible for approximately 63% of the cases worldwide, while an intestinal and hepatic form caused by *S. mansoni* accounts for another 35% (Table 3.1).[11] Less than 1% of the global burden of schistosomiasis results from the Cold War warrior *S. japonicum*.[1] Almost all of the people infected with schistosomiasis live in Africa, with 29 African nations each harboring 1 million or more cases (Color Plate 5).[1] Outside Africa, only the nations of Brazil and Yemen have 1 million or more cases of schistosomiasis.[1] In Brazil and elsewhere in the Americas,

Table 3.1 The major human schistosomes

Species	Length as adult	Disease	No. of cases worldwide	Major geographic locations
S. haematobium	10–20 mm (0.4–0.8 in.)	Urinary and urogenital schistosomiasis	130 million	Africa, Middle East
S. mansoni	6–17 mm (0.2–0.7 in.)	Intestinal and hepatic schistosomiasis	73 million	Africa, Middle East, Americas
S. japonicum and *S. mekongi*	12–26 mm (0.5–1.0 in.)	Intestinal and hepatic schistosomiasis	2 million	China, the Philippines, Southeast Asia

Schistosomiasis

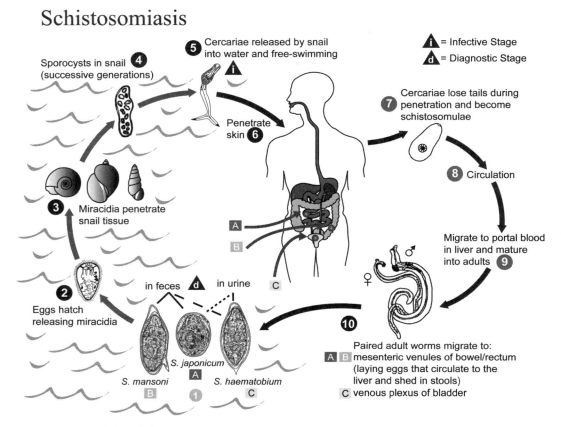

Figure 3.1 The life cycle of human schistosomes (Public Health Image Library, CDC [http://phil.cdc.gov]).

S. mansoni infection was likely introduced by a flourishing slave trade with sub-Saharan Africa that began in the 1600s.[12]

Humans contract schistosomiasis through freshwater contact with free-swimming cercariae (Fig. 3.1). Therefore, poor rural populations whose everyday activities involve fishing, bathing, or swimming in schistosome-contaminated waters or working in agricultural areas irrigated by contaminated waters are at the highest risk of infection.[10,13] An estimated 779 million people in developing countries live near either irrigated agricultural fields or dam reservoirs, where the risk of acquiring schistosmiasis is the highest.[1]

Schistosome cercariae have a forked tail that allows them to swim and ultimately to directly penetrate human skin. Following skin penetration, the cercariae lose their tail and undergo a number of biochemical changes that allow them to resist attack by the human immune system. The larval schistosomes (also known as schistosomulae) migrate through the lungs and over a period of approximately 4 to 6 weeks make their way to the portal vein of the liver, where they mature into adult male and female schistosomes. The paired worms ultimately migrate to their final destination, which for *S. haematobium*, the cause of urinary tract schistosomiasis, is the small veins that drain the bladder, while *S. mansoni* and *S. japonicum* live in the mesenteric veins that drain the intestine. While living in the blood vessels, the adult schistosomes feed on blood, breaking down the hemoglobin components by using enzymes similar to those found in hookworms. Through evolution, the adult male and female schistosomes living in the bloodstream have developed remarkable mechanisms for masking their identity, including the accretion of host molecules on their surface. In this way, the schistosomes avoid attack by antibodies and cells of the human immune system.

The female worms subsequently produce hundreds of eggs daily.[13] In order to continue the schistosome life cycle, the eggs ultimately require a mechanism to exit from the body. In the case of hookworm infection and other soil-transmitted helminth infections in which the parasites live in the gastrointestinal tract, the feces provide a straightforward path for the eggs to escape into the environment. In contrast, schistosome eggs have a more formidable challenge because they are present in the human blood vessels. As shown in Fig. 3.2, schistosome eggs are equipped with an ominous-appearing spine that permits them to bore their way through the blood vessels and then into either the bladder or intestine from the outside. Through a combination of mechanical boring and the release of tissue-dissolving enzymes, the eggs gain access to

Figure 3.2 Spined eggs of *S. haematobium* (top) and *S. mansoni* (bottom) (Public Health Image Library, CDC [http://phil.cdc.gov]).

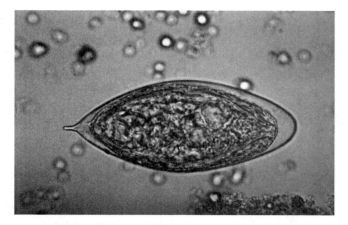

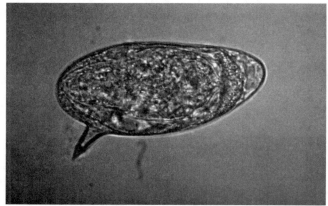

either the lumen of the bladder or the intestine; they exit the body in urine or feces, respectively. When deposited in freshwater, the eggs live for about a week. They hatch and give rise to free-swimming ciliated forms known as miracidia, which seek out a suitable snail species. Upon entry into the appropriate snail, each miracidium can give rise to multiple progeny through asexual reproduction. Eventually, these progeny develop into cercariae that exit the snail.[13]

Unfortunately, egg migration through human body tissues is not an efficient process, so many eggs become trapped in either the bladder (*S. haematobium*) or intestine and liver (*S. mansoni* and *S. japonicum*). The trapped eggs cause mechanical damage and the rupture of small blood vessels, which lead to bleeding and the appearance of blood in either urine or feces. The eggs also trigger an inflammatory response composed of masses of human white cells and other host-derived components (known as granulomas), which can obstruct urine or blood flow. Because schistosomes can live for years in the small veins of the bladder and intestine, their constant release of eggs is associated with chronic blood loss leading to anemia, as well as damage to the bladder and kidneys (*S. haematobium*) or to the intestine and liver (*S. mansoni*). The combination of long-standing anemia, inflammation, and target organ damage causes growth retardation, undernutrition, and cognitive delays in children, as well as chronic abdominal pain, exercise intolerance, poor school performance, and reduced work capacity.[13,14] Anemia and chronic inflammation also partially account for the developmental delays occurring in chronic pediatric soil-transmitted helminth infections.

Sub-Saharan Africa bears the greatest burden of disease caused by the schistsosomes and almost all of the cases of *S. haematobium* infection. Color Plate 6 shows several children, each holding a cup of his or her reddened urine (schistosomiasis is sometimes known locally as red-water fever, as well as snail fever). Endemic hematuria from schistosomiasis was first recorded in 1798 by a Western physician, J. Renoult, a French army surgeon who accompanied Napoleon on his invasion of Egypt.[2] Just as hookworm causes chronic blood loss in the intestine, leading to anemia, the chronic blood loss resulting from *S. haematobium* egg deposition in the bladder is a significant cause of anemia in Africa, particularly among adolescent children, who on average harbor larger numbers of schistosomes than do any other age group.[11] We saw previously how chronic intestinal blood loss and anemia resulting from hookworm were associated with physical and mental delays in children. For urinary schistosomiasis, the anemia results not only from urinary blood loss but also from other factors, including chronic inflammation. These processes also contribute to inhibition of physical and mental growth for the child. Other important contributors to the morbidity of urinary schistosomiasis are the inflammatory granulomas that develop in the bladder. Severe bladder wall pathology occurs in an estimated 18 million people in Africa.[15] When the bladder granulomas coalesce, they can obstruct urine flow and cause distension of the ureter and kidneys. This condition is known as hydronephrosis and occurs in approximately 20 million people in Africa as a result of *S. haematobium* infection.[15] Long-standing hydronephrosis can lead to renal failure; this progression probably accounts for a significant number of the estimated 280,000 deaths from schistosomiasis.[15] Another major consequence of chronic *S. haematobium* infection is its ability to predispose people to acquiring an unusual form of bladder cancer. Whereas most bladder carcinomas in the industrialized world are adenocarcinomas, *S. haematobium* infection is associated with a unique squamous cell carcinoma of the bladder. It is conjectured that the schistosome granulomas in the bladder may increase the exposure of the bladder epithelium to environmental carcinogens.[13] Still another important component of the morbidity of *S. haematobium* infection is involvement of the female reproductive tract. Up to 75% of women with this form of schistosomiasis exhibit lesions in the vulva, vagina, cervix, and uterus. Genital schistosomiasis lesions recently have been linked to a threefold increase in the transmission of HIV/AIDS in Zimbabwe and presumably elsewhere in sub-Saharan Africa.[16] From these and similar studies, there is considerable interest in looking at schistosomiasis control and prevention efforts in terms of their impact on HIV transmission in rural areas of Africa.[16]

S. mansoni is also a significant cause of intestinal and liver pathology in sub-Saharan Africa and Brazil. The presence of eggs and granulomas in the intestinal wall, usually of the large intestine and rectum, is associated with bleeding and diarrhea, as well as with loss of appetite, while liver granulomas can cause inflammation and liver enlargement (hence the term big-belly disease).[13] Chronic schistosomiasis of the liver can progress to fibrosis, splenic enlargement, and bleeding from the esophagus. Occasionally, severe bleeding can result in death. An estimated 8.5 million cases of liver disease result from *S. mansoni* infection in sub-Saharan Africa.[15]

Although snail control was the major tool used to effect an almost 10-fold reduction in the prevalence of *S. japonicum* infection in China, this approach has not been an efficient or very effective means for controlling either *S. haematobium* or *S. mansoni* in Africa and elsewhere. Failed efforts to control snails environmentally reflect the unique biology of the snail intermediate hosts of *S. haematobium* and *S. mansoni* as well as the epidemiology of these forms of schistosomiasis. In addition, the environmental toxicities of molluscicides preclude their constant and widespread use. Even in China, snail control has not been successful in eliminating the last remaining 840,000 cases in the Yangtze River valley.[6]

We saw previously (in chapter 2) how mass drug administration of benzimidazole anthelmintics is beginning to have an impact on the global burden of disease caused by soil-transmitted helminth infections. Today, the most effective means of controlling schistosome infections is mass drug administration of praziquantel to affected and at-risk human populations. Developed at Bayer, praziquantel was shown to be effective against all forms of schistosomiasis in multicenter trials, as evidenced by schistosome egg reductions or outright cures.[10] Treatment of schistosome-infected children with praziquantel results in a number of health benefits similar to those experienced by children with soil-transmitted helminth infections who are treated with either albendazole or mebendazole, including improvements in growth and physical fitness, as well as reduction of anemia.[11] In addition, multiple treatments with praziquantel can sometimes reverse both urinary tract and liver pathology, particularly if children receive these treatments early in their lives.[11] Building on these breakthrough medical observations were the low-cost synthesis and production methods for manufacturing generic praziquantel developed by the Korean pharmaceutical company Shin Poong. These manufacturing improvements have dramatically reduced the price of the drug, possibly by as much as 90%.[10] As a result, by the 1990s, it became possible to launch praziquantel mass treatment programs for schistosomiasis in several middle-income countries, including Brazil, China, Egypt, Morocco, the Philippines, Saudi Arabia, and Tunisia, as well as Puerto Rico.[10,13,17] Several of these initiatives were funded by the World Bank. Praziquantel mass drug administration in these countries has been largely successful, particularly in Morocco and Puerto Rico, where the disease is close to being eliminated (zero transmission) partly because of parallel poverty reduction measures that were enacted.[10]

Previously (in chapter 2), we learned how in 2001, the 54th World Health Assembly adopted a resolution calling for treatment with a benzimidazole anthelmintic drug of at least 75% of school-age children at risk of acquiring schistosomiasis and soil-transmitted helminth infections by 2010.[11] Based on the experiences and successes of mass drug administration of praziquantel, the resolution was written to include this drug along with either albendazole or mebendazole for treating school-age children (see the Partners for Parasite Control website [http://who.int/wormcontrol/]). In many regions of the developing world, especially in sub-Saharan Africa and Brazil, it is common for children to be polyparasitized with both soil-transmitted helminths (especially hookworm) and schistosomes,[18] so that they could benefit from combination therapy of a benzimidazole anthelmintic and praziquantel. In response to the 2001 World Health Assembly resolution, the Bill and Melinda Gates Foundation funded the Schistosomiasis Control Initiative (SCI), a public-private partnership established by Alan Fenwick at Imperial College London (http://www.schisto.org) to begin implementation of praziquantel (together with either single-dose albendazole or mebendazole) mass drug administration in sub-Saharan Africa, where the disease burden is greatest. Previously, Fenwick had acquired a wide-ranging experience in large-scale control of schistosomiasis through his leadership in World Bank- and U.S. Agency for International Development-funded projects in Egypt and Sudan.

Working through the National Control Programs of six sub-Saharan African countries—Burkina Faso, Mali, Niger, Tanzania, Uganda, and Zambia—together with the World Health Organization, the SCI facilitates once-yearly praziquantel treatments using donated generic praziquantel from MedPharm and other sources. SCI operates through algorithms based on the schistosomiasis prevalence determined in local school surveys.[17] The number of praziqantel tablets administered to each individual is based on an easy-to-use height pole that approximates a dose of 40 mg of drug per kg of body weight, and the delivery and distribution of praziquantel are carried out in health centers, in schools, or through community-based drug distributors.[10]

To date, SCI has made some impressive public health gains, scoring significant and dramatic reductions in the prevalence of schistosomiasis.[17,19] In each of the six SCI target countries, national plans have been developed and are now being implemented. To date, approximately 1 million people have been treated in the three West African countries, and over 2 million people have been treated in Uganda.[10] Presently, Uganda conducts annual dewormings with praziquantel and a benzimidazole anthelmintic on designated child health days, and now similar child health day programs in conjunction with the World Food Programme are under way in Tanzania and Zambia.[10] Through additional funding from Legatum and Geneva Global, SCI, in collaboration with the Global Network for Neglected Tropical Diseases, is about to launch new programs in Rwanda and possibly elsewhere. Such efforts have also led to improvements in anemia and other features of schistosomiasis morbidity. Important future avenues of investigation include the potential effects of praziquantel mass drug administration on reducing HIV/AIDS transmission as well as the effect on schistosomiasis and anemia in pregnancy.[16]

There are a number of important but still unanswered questions about the impact of praziquantel mass drug administration on sustainable poverty reduction in developing countries. Present-day population-based approaches with praziquantel are focused on reducing the morbidity of this condition in areas where high-intensity infections and serious urogenital, intestinal, and liver morbidities are present. However, it is unclear whether mass treatment will also reduce transmission and prevent reinfection in the community.[20] This uncertainty is a serious concern, since ongoing low levels of schistosomiasis reinfection could lead to subtle but persistent clinical problems, including anemia, growth stunting, and diminished productive capacities.[20] In addition, there are potential worries that frequent and periodic use of praziquantel could lead to anthelmintic drug resistance.[17] These issues have prompted some nascent efforts to develop alternative or complementary control tools for schistosomiasis, just as they have for human hookworm infection. These activities include exploration of new drug development, including the antimalarial artemisinin, artemether, which also exhibits antischistosomal properties.[21] Still another approach has been efforts to develop a recombinant vaccine for schistosomiasis (discussed in chapter 11).[22] However, our major approach to schistosomiasis control still relies on mass drug administration of praziquantel or of praziquantel and albendazole or mebendazole in areas of schistosomiasis and soil-transmitted helminth coinfection. We will further explore (in chapter 10) how these treatments might link with mass drug administrations for other neglected tropical diseases, including lymphatic filariasis, onchocerciasis, and trachoma.

Summary Points: Schistosomiasis

- Significant impact on the modern history of China and Egypt
- One of the most common and clinically important human helminth infections
- Schistosomiasis is a waterborne infectious disease transmitted by a snail intermediate host.
- Approximately 207 million cases worldwide, with 97% of the infections in Africa
- Children and adolescents at highest risk. All forms of chronic schistosomiasis are associated with anemia, undernutrition and growth impairments, poor school performance, and reduced productive capacity.
- Urinary schistosomiasis caused by *S. haematobium* accounts for approximately two-thirds of the schistosome infections in Africa. This form is responsible for hematuria, urogenital pathology, and squamous cell carcinoma of the bladder. Genital lesions increase the risk of HIV/AIDS transmission.
- Intestinal and liver schistosomiasis caused by *S. mansoni* accounts for approximately one-third of the cases in Africa and 1 million cases of schistosomiasis in Brazil. This form is responsible for bloody diarrhea, abdominal pain, and liver involvement (hepatomegaly and fibrosis).
- The major approach to control of schistosomiasis today is mass drug administration of praziquantel. It has led to the near elimination of schistosomiasis in some middle-income countries and to significant morbidity reductions in some sub-Saharan African countries.

The Filarial Infections: Lymphatic Filariasis (Elephantiasis) and Dracunculiasis (Guinea Worm)

> *Moving from the jungle was a native with elephantiasis…pushing a rude wheelbarrow before him. In the barrow rested his scrotum, a monstrous growth that…weighed more than 70 pounds and tied him a prisoner to his barrow.*
>
> JAMES MICHENER, TALES OF THE SOUTH PACIFIC[1]

Elephantiasis is the most severe and dramatic complication of lymphatic filariasis (LF), a chronic infection caused primarily by the filarial parasite *Wuchereria bancrofti*. Dracunculiasis is another chronic infection caused by a filaria-like parasite, *Dracunculus medinensis*, also known as the guinea worm. Although both LF and dracunculiasis are still serious public health problems in the developing world, we are much farther along in our global efforts to control these ancient scourges than we are with the soil-transmitted helminth (STH) infections or schistosomiasis. For LF, mass drug administration is progressing to the point where we believe that there is a real possibility that this infection could be one day eliminated. We are on the verge of eradicating dracunculiasis. Our use of the terms elimination and eradication is deliberate. Elimination refers to reduction of the prevalence of an infection to the point where transmission has been interrupted but ongoing public health control measures must still be maintained. Eradication refers to the disappearance of naturally occurring infection to the point where public health intervention measures can be halted. To date, smallpox is the only disease ever to be eradicated.

Although filariae are nematodes, they bear little resemblance to the STHs described in chapter 2. As adult worms, the filariae grow to enormous lengths

Table 4.1 Major filariae or filaria-like parasites of humans

Disease	Alternative name	Estimated global prevalence (no of cases); location	Parasite	Location of adult parasite in humans	Length as adults (male and female)	Arthropod vector
LF	Elephantiasis	120 million; India, East Asia and Pacific, Africa, Americas	*W. bancrofti* (major); *Brugia malayi* and *Brugia timori* (minor)	Lymphatics, genitals	4–10 cm (1.5–4 in.)	Mosquito
Onchocerciasis	River blindness	37 million; Africa	*Onchocerca volvulus*	Subcutaneous tissues	2–50 cm (1–20 in.)	Blackfly
Loiasis	African eye worm	13 million; Africa	*Loa loa*	Subcutaneous tissues	3–7 cm (1–3 in.)	Tabanid fly
Dracunculiasis	Guinea worm	1.01 million; Africa	*D. medinensis*	Subcutaneous tissues	4–100 cm (1.5–40 in.)	Copepod
Heartworm	Dog heart-worm	Rare parasite of humans	*Dirofilaria immitis*	Heart	12–30 cm (5–12 in.)	Mosquito

(sometimes a yard or more) in various body tissues such as the lymphatics, genitals, or subcutaneous tissues, instead of in the gastrointestinal tract. Moreover, they are transmitted by the bites of arthropod vectors rather than through soil contamination. Table 4.1 lists the major filarial parasites of humans, the diseases that they cause, their geographic prevalence and location, and their arthropod vectors. I include dog heartworm on this list, because many pet owners in "the North" are already familiar with this parasite. This chapter will consider LF and dracunculiasis, while onchocerciasis, another filarial infection, will be discussed together with trachoma (in chapter 5) as major causes of blindness.

LF

Ancient records of LF include a statue with swollen limbs of Egyptian Pharaoh Mentuhotep II from 2000 BCE and descriptions by the Persian physician Avicenna (Ibn Sina, 981–1037), who distinguished this disease from leprosy.[1] Today, most of the world's 120 million LF cases occur among the poorest people living in either India or sub-Saharan Africa, although large numbers of cases still occur in Southeast Asia, on the Pacific islands, and in some tropical areas of the Americas (especially Haiti, the Dominican Republic, and northeastern Brazil) (Color Plate 7).[2]

The adult *W. bancrofti* worms that cause 90% of the cases of LF (the other infections are caused by worms of the genus *Brugia*) live in human lymphatics (vessel-like structures that parallel and feed into the bloodstream) mostly located in the inguinal region (groin) and genitals. The adult female worms attain up to 4 in. in length and resemble a coiled-up piece of string or angel-hair pasta. How and why the adult worms develop in the lymphatics versus other sites are not known. However, since the lymphatics are a rich source of antibodies and cells of the immune system, it is all the more remarkable that the adult filarial worms could survive for up to several years in what is arguably one of the most inhospitable places for foreign pathogens imaginable.

After mating, the female filarial worm, like the STHs and the schistosomes, produces a large number of embryos contained within eggshells (Fig. 4.1). However, the embryos of *W. bancrofti* do not take an egg-like shape but instead take an elongated shape, resembling tiny worms measuring roughly 0.25 mm in length. These so-called "*microfilariae*" migrate to the bloodstream, where ultimately they can be ingested by an appropriate species of female mosquito feeding on blood. It was Sir Patrick Manson, often considered the father of modern tropical medicine, who in 1877 first elucidated some of the fundamental aspects of the life cycle of *W. bancrofti*, including its transmission via mosquitoes.[1]

Figure 4.1 Life cycle of *W. bancrofti* (Public Health Image Library, CDC [http://phil.cdc.gov]).

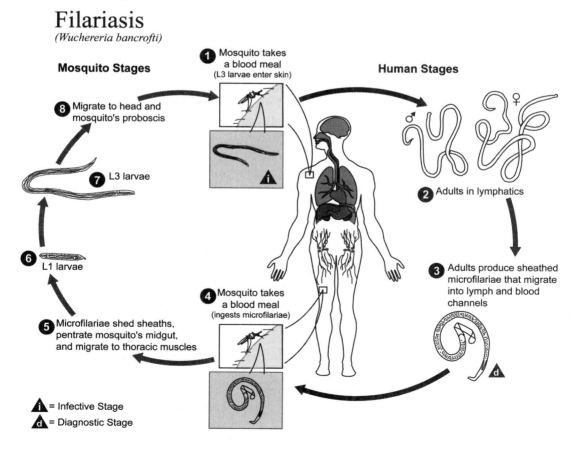

Filariasis
(Wuchereria bancrofti)

Mosquito Stages

1 Mosquito takes a blood meal (L3 larvae enter skin)

Human Stages

8 Migrate to head and mosquito's proboscis

7 L3 larvae

6 L1 larvae

2 Adults in lymphatics

5 Microfilariae shed sheaths, pentrate mosquito's midgut, and migrate to thoracic muscles

4 Mosquito takes a blood meal (ingests microfilariae)

3 Adults produce sheathed microfilariae that migrate into lymph and blood channels

i = Infective Stage

d = Diagnostic Stage

Once in the mosquito, the microfilariae develop, penetrate the stomach wall, and after about 10 to 12 days develop into larval stages that are capable of infecting humans the next time that the mosquito bites. In sub-Saharan Africa and elsewhere, the same mosquito species that transmit malaria also transmit LF. However, *W. bancrofti* is far less selective, so several different genera of mosquitoes are capable of hosting infective larvae and transmitting the infection. The infective larvae that migrate to the mouth parts of the mosquito can penetrate human skin. Possibly this presentation occurs through a puncture site generated by the insect. Then over a period of months, the larvae migrate to their final destination in the lymphatics, where they grow into adult worms. The adult worms can live for extraordinarily long periods, often for 8 years or more.[3] This life span is amazing for an invertebrate but not unusual for parasitic worms. Why parasitic worms tend to live so much longer than their free-living counterparts is still a mystery.

In fact, there are a number of mysteries about the life history of *W. bancrofti* and the disease that it causes. Among them is the curious observation that over a 24-h period, the microfilariae tend to accumulate in the blood only at certain hours. In most of the world, *W. bancrofti* microfilariae appear in the victim's circulation at night, when the mosquitoes are biting the most. In some cases, the timing is very precise so that microfilariae appear between 10 p.m. and 4 a.m. Since older methods for diagnosing LF required sampling the blood to look for microfilariae under a microscope, establishing a diagnosis of LF used to require operating clinics in the dead of night.[4] Like so many NTDs, LF is understudied and we still do not understand the physiological basis by which the microfilariae exhibit the unusual circadian rhythm known as nocturnal periodicity. Of interest is the observation that it is sometimes possible to reverse nocturnal periodicity by altering the sleep-wake cycle of an infected individual; this observation suggests that somehow the human host trains the microfilariae to keep up with the human schedule. Yet another mystery is how the adult *W. bancrofti* worms can survive for 8 years or more in a part of the body where they are practically bathed in host antibody and immune attacking cells. The immune evasion tactics by the adult worms are still not well understood, but there are some data to indicate that they somehow can manipulate the human immune system in order to make the host tolerant of their presence.[5]

We also do not understand well the sequence of events by which a person infected with LF can progress from having no symptoms to having horrible and disfiguring elephantiasis. Adding to the complexity is the observation that some patients can remain asymptomatic and never develop further complications. To our best knowledge, the pathologic sequence of events leading to disfigurement is initiated when the adult *W. bancrofti* worms dilate the lymphatic vessels where they reside.[6] In some cases this vessel dilation phenomenon (known as lymphangiectasia) occurs because the adult worms cause lymphatic obstruction, but blockage is not always a requirement. Lymphangiectasia often occurs silently, or in some cases it can be seen by applying an ultrasound probe to the skin surface in the region of the groin. When ultrasonography is done, it is frequently possible to see worms writhing within the dilated lymphatics. The so-called "filarial dance sign" is one of the first indications that someone has acquired a new filarial infection, and it is one of the first signs of infection in children and young adolescents as they grow up in a part of the world where LF is endemic.

Late in the lymphangiectasia phase of the infection, the filarial worms reach the upper limit of their life span and start to die. In a village where LF is endemic, parasite death typically starts to occur by the time infected children are well into adolescence. However, unlike many infections with which we are familiar—such as bacterial and viral infections, in which it is a desired goal for either our host immune response or antimicrobial agents administered by a physician to kill the offending pathogens—the death of adult filarial worms in vthe lymphatics of adolescents is not necessarily a good thing to happen. Instead, it is believed that the dead and dying worms lose their immunological masking properties, which results in a stimulus for the human immune response to release a cascade of cytokine inflammatory mediators. For the patient, the resulting cytokine storm produces fever and swelling of the lymphatics. Concurrently, secondary bacterial infections occur, with the parasites themselves contributing some of the bacteria (we will see in chapters 5 and 11 how some filarial parasites are naturally infected with bacterial endosymbionts). Our present thinking about LF is that the new inflammation against the dead parasites and the accompanying bacterial infections combine to initiate the first steps in a disease process lasting years, one subsequently leading to the characteristic lymph and genital deformities of elephantiasis.[6,7] The long time required for this series of events to unfold largely explains why elephantiasis usually occurs only in adulthood.

The health and socioeconomic impact of LF for the poorest people of India, Africa, and elsewhere is huge. The initial filarial fevers of adolescents are associated with enlarged, warm and painful lymph nodes, and males experience tenderness and swelling in their scrotum, which is sometimes associated with hydrocele, an accumulation of fluid in the sac surrounding the testicles. Some patients develop lymphedema, i.e., edema and swelling of the legs and scrotum, with thickening and loss of skin elasticity. As lymphedema progresses, the limb and overlying skin begin to resemble an elephant's leg. The affected leg can become ulcerated and infected with bacteria.[6,7] Thus, LF exhibits a wide spectrum of disease, ranging from asymptomatic cases to filarial fevers and swellings to lymphedema and elephantiasis. Of the estimated 120 million people with LF, approximately 43 million suffer from hydrocele, lymphedema, and other evidence of severe LF disease.[8]

While the health impact of these pathologic changes is fairly obvious, like many NTDs, LF has equally serious economic and social effects. Although death from LF is rare, the disease is nevertheless devastating because it strikes otherwise young and productive adults. In males, LF is a particular threat for agricultural laborers, usually of extremely modest means, who either are incapacitated with filarial fevers or are forced to give up their jobs because of their hydrocele or lymphedema. Myrtle Perera, a social worker from Sri Lanka, has extensively studied young coconut pickers who are no longer able to climb trees because of their hydroceles.[9] In one case, a worker commented that his hydrocele was as big as the coconuts he was picking.[9] Similarly, in Haiti, women with lymphedema frequently cannot participate in market trading, their major form of economic activity, while in northern Ghana, the incapacitating episodes of acute lymphangitis often reach their peak in rainy season, ordinarily a time of maximal agricultural activity.[9] Throughout the regions of the developing world where LF is endemic, it is a common practice for afflicted workers to change their trade to one that requires fewer physically demanding tasks in order to accommodate their disabilities.[9]

K. D. Ramaiah of India has conducted economic analyses of the impact of LF pathology on worker productivity and has identified a huge effect: the annual loss of US$842 million, almost 0.1% of India's GNP (gross national product).[9,10] In Orissa State, India, chronic LF patients lose a total of 68 days of work per year, equivalent to 19% of the total working time of the year, and spend 2% of their annual wages on treatment.[9,10] Another important impact, although one less easy to quantify, is the stigma of having LF. The example of the woman who lost her job because of LF's stigmatizing aspects was illustrated in chapter 1. In addition, the stigma of hydrocele and elephantiasis is today causing millions of young men to hide their condition for years and prevent them from seeking medical attention.

Figure 4.2 presents pictures of Stephen J. Hawking and Mao Zedong. They are connected in a very interesting way by LF and the prospects for controlling it. While almost everyone has heard of Professor Hawking, the great cosmologist and father of the Big Bang theory, far fewer know that his father, Frank Hawking, was a parasitologist who studied LF and traveled widely in order to develop new approaches to its control. During the 1950s and 1960s, the senior Hawking made important contributions to the development and testing of drugs that target *W. bancrofti*, including a compound known as diethylcarbamazine, often abbreviated as DEC.[11] Hawking and others demonstrated that DEC was highly effective against the microfilarial stages of *W. bancrofti* but much less so against the adult stages. DEC is now widely administered in the treatment of LF worldwide. But since all the pathology resulting from LF is caused by adult worms and not by the microfilariae, what would then be the rationale of targeting the microfilariae?

During World War II, LF was a major health problem for U.S. troops fighting in the South Pacific. It was estimated that approximately 38,300 U.S. naval personnel were exposed during the war, about one-third of whom developed filarial fevers.[12] These concerns led groups of American and other scientists to take a greater interest in the problem of LF and possible approaches for controlling it. Shortly after the end of World War II, John F. Kessel of UCLA and his colleagues working in Tahiti began looking at the impact of mass administration of DEC to infected populations. They demonstrated that, by administering a drug that lowers the number of microfilariae among an entire village, it would be possible to interrupt the transmission of LF even if it did not directly reduce the immediate suffering from the disease.[13] In order to make this process more efficient, Frank Hawking pioneered the concept of fortifying dietary

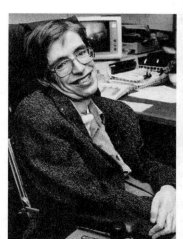
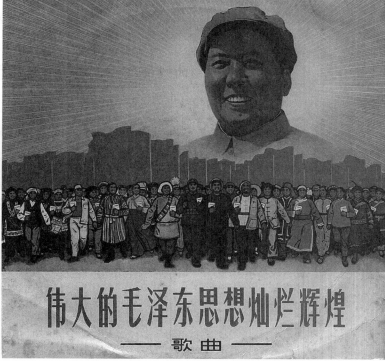

Figure 4.2 What do Stephen Hawking and Mao Zedong have in common?

salt with DEC.[14] DEC is a highly stable compound, and even cooking does not destroy the drug. Therefore, instead of iodizing the salt, Hawking proposed DEC'ing it, and he began administering the medicated salt in food in order to reduce microfilarial loads among the population. The DEC-fortified salt study provided an important proof of concept that this approach could be an important weapon in the fight against endemic LF. However, it took the Chinese to apply it on an almost unimaginable scale.

While Hawking was working in Brazil, on the other side of the world, the People's Republic of China under the leadership of Mao Zedong was suffering some of the highest rates of LF. Indeed, the life cycle of LF was discovered by Sir Patrick Manson in the city of Amoy (renamed Xiamen) in Fujian Province on China's coast. Manson's landmark study demonstrated for the first time that a human infection could be transmitted by a mosquito vector. This observation laid the foundation for subsequent studies by Sir Ronald Ross in India, who demonstrated that mosquitoes transmitted malaria. In 1976 in Shandong Province, also on the coast of China (roughly 100 years following Manson's discoveries), DEC-medicated salt was administered to almost 40,000 people for 6 months, with a resulting dramatic reduction in the prevalence of LF as determined by the numbers of microfilariae in blood.[15] Studies such as this one were followed with efforts to scale up LF control for all of China's major provinces at risk for the disease. As a result of blanket coverage with DEC-fortified salt, today the People's Republic of China represents one of the first large nations to have successfully eliminated LF, which it did under Mao Zedong's leadership. Subsequently, widespread use of DEC-fortified salt resulted in the elimination or near elimination of *W. bancrofti* infection from Brazil, Japan, Tanzania, and Taiwan,[16] while mass administration of the drug as tablets has over a period of 5 years resulted in the elimination of LF from Egypt.[17] For some of these countries, mosquito control was a critical adjunct for LF elimination efforts, while in the case of the Solomon Islands, vector control was sufficient for LF elimination.[18] In most of sub-Saharan Africa, the drug ivermectin is used in place of DEC, because of its better safety profile in patients who are coinfected with onchocerciasis (the widespread use of ivermectin in Africa is discussed in chapter 5).

A number of factors, both biological and social, provide great optimism that LF elimination efforts through mass drug administration could be extended worldwide.[19] They include the observations that a single dose of either DEC or ivermectin can reduce the number of blood-circulating microfilariae for up to 1 year, that humans are the only significant reservoir of infection caused by *W. bancrofti*, and that mosquito transmission is highly inefficient. It is certainly less efficient than it is for malaria and therefore more easily interrupted by vector control methods (including bed nets). In addition, we have the proof of concept that it has been possible to eliminate LF in some countries. Based on these assumptions, in 1997 the World Health Assembly (WHA) adopted a resolution to eliminate LF as a public health problem by 2020.[20] The major components of the LF elimination strategy follow: first, interrupt LF transmission by using one of two single-dose, two-drug treatment regimens, either DEC plus albendazole or ivermectin plus albendazole (albendazole is added in order to forestall the emergence of drug resistance), with once-yearly administration of these two drug regimens in order to achieve four to six annual consecutive rounds of high coverage; and second, reduce the existing morbidity of LF, particularly filarial fevers, hydrocele, and lymphedema and/or elephantiasis, with an emphasis on hygiene, skin care, and simple surgery.[19] Thus, mass drug administration for LF of either ivermectin and albendazole or DEC and albendazole joins other mass treatments for STH infections (using albendazole or mebendazole) and for schistosomiasis (using praziquantel) as major approaches to global NTD control.

In response to the WHA resolution, the health ministers from all the countries in the Pacific region agreed to meet with the WHO Western Pacific Regional Office (WPRO) in order to establish PacELF for the elimination of LF in the region through mass drug administration, with each country adopting its own such strategy.[18] After five rounds of mass drug administration, LF has now been eliminated on the Cook Islands and in Niue and Samoa. However, outside the Pacific region, LF remains endemic in 76 countries, and most of the countries in sub-Saharan Africa have no well-established LF elimination programs under way.

In 2000, the Global Alliance to Eliminate LF (GAELF) (http://www.filaria.org) was formed to support a global program for helping to ensure elimination by 2020. Among the areas of emphasis, GAELF is working to facilitate establishment of programs in Africa and parts of Asia where infrastructure is lacking. GAELF also has as a major goal the alleviation of the physical, social and economic hardships of individuals who have LF-induced disabilities. The Secretariat of GAELF is based at the Liverpool School of Tropical Medicine, with David H. Molyneux as the present director. Molyneux also runs an LF Support Centre in Liverpool. His work is being facilitated by the investigation of a number of operational research questions by Eric Ottesen and his associates at a second LF Support Center based at the Task Force for Child Survival and Development in Atlanta, GA.

By the end of 2004, it was estimated that a total of 248 million people had been treated through mass drug administration of DEC or ivermectin. While this accomplishment is impressive, it has been estimated that between 62 and 79% of the world's at-risk population (roughly 600 to 800 million people) remains untreated.[19] Moreover, only 6% of the world's at-risk population has received two-drug regimens. These observations, coupled with concerns that there are inadequate financial resources for the purchase and administration of DEC as well as funds for monitoring, evaluation, and operational research,[19,20] suggest that even though we have excellent tools in hand, and even though the biological and social features of LF are favorable for elimination, it is not at all clear that, at our present pace, we will meet the WHA elimination target by 2020. Additional hurdles include the fact that most of the 600 to 800 million people who need access to treatment are at the bottom of the economic scale and therefore politically voiceless.[19] Adding even further to these social and political barriers to mass drug administration is the stigmatizing element of LF, which means that many people with the disease are hidden from view. Stigma prevents accurate assessments of disease burden and access to essential medicines. Later, we will see how, through linking LF control with other NTD control efforts, the Global Network for NTDs could increase the efficiencies of ongoing LF elimination efforts as a means for achieving the ambitious targets set by the WHA.

Dracunculiasis (guinea worm infection)

Except for about 25,000 remaining cases, mostly in Sudan and Ghana, human guinea worm infection has been practically eradicated from the planet. Guinea worm is thought to have been the Biblical "fiery red serpent" attacking Israelites in the desert after their exodus from Egypt, with therapies describing methods for extracting it found in Egyptian medical papyri.[1] By 1986, it was estimated that approximately 3.5 million cases of guinea worm infection occurred among the poorest people in Africa, the Middle East, and Asia. However, through an extraordinary program of public health control and advocacy, the Carter Center in cooperation with the CDC, UNICEF, and WHO has led a 20-year-long global dracunculiasis eradication program, which has so far resulted in a 99% reduction in incidence of the disease.[21]

The guinea worm, *D. medinensis*, is not a true filarial worm like *W. bancrofti*, but they have a number of similarities. The adult worms grow to up to a yard in length (females are longer than males) and inhabit the tissues of the legs and feet, just under the skin. Occasionally, they are located in other body parts. The adult female has evolved an interesting way of getting her larval offspring into the environment by producing substances that create a blister under the skin. The blister is under pressure, and when an individual immerses his leg in water, the blister ruptures. During this process, the female adult worm discharges a milky-white substance containing thousands of immature *D. medinensis* larvae. Larval discharge and release can continue for days. The larvae survive in fresh water and develop further after being swallowed by a small crustacean called a copepod. Humans then become infected when they swallow unfiltered or unboiled water containing copepods (Fig. 4.3). After ingestion, the copepod is digested by gastric acid, but the infective guinea worm larvae survive this insult. The larvae released in the human gastrointestinal tract penetrate the human gut and over a period of

Figure 4.3 The life cycle of the guinea worm (Public Health Image Library, CDC [http://phil.cdc.gov]).

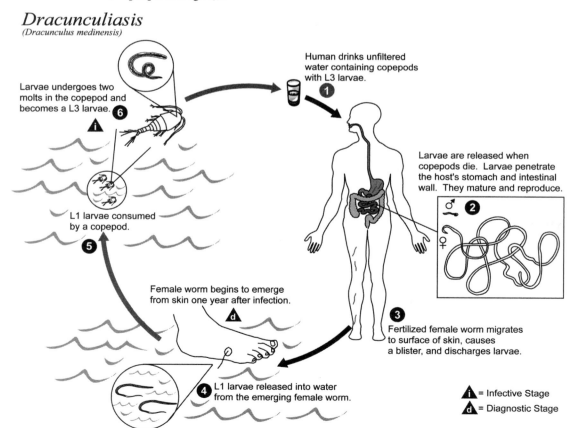

Dracunculiasis
(Dracunculus medinensis)

Larvae undergoes two molts in the copepod and becomes a L3 larvae. **6**

Human drinks unfiltered water containing copepods with L3 larvae. 1

Larvae are released when copepods die. Larvae penetrate the host's stomach and intestinal wall. They mature and reproduce. 2

L1 larvae consumed by a copepod. **5**

Female worm begins to emerge from skin one year after infection.

Fertilized female worm migrates to surface of skin, causes a blister, and discharges larvae. 3

4 L1 larvae released into water from the emerging female worm.

= Infective Stage

= Diagnostic Stage

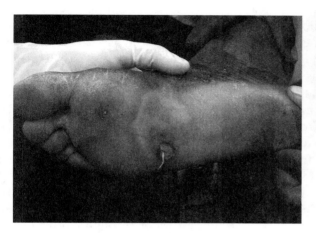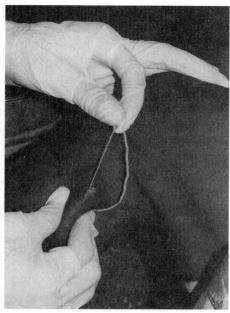

Figure 4.4 Clinical infection with guinea worm (courtesy The Carter Center).

several months make their way to the connective tissue of the legs, where they sexually mature and mate.

Almost all of the symptoms of guinea worm infection result from the presence of the adult worm residing in the legs (Fig. 4.4). The blister produced by female worms is painful and can cause a burning sensation. These processes can go on for 2 or 3 months, during which time the individual is often incapacitated and unable to work.[21] In some cases, the pain can continue for 1 to 2 years. In the resource-poor settings where guinea worm occurs, it is common for the ulcer that results from the ruptured blister to become infected with bacteria; both secondary bacterial infections and sometimes even tetanus are well-known complications. When the worm is located near joints (commonly the ankle joint), the inflammation can cause arthritis, which can be severe at times.

Prior to large-scale control efforts, it was common for entire villages to be affected simultaneously. When guinea worm infection epidemics struck during a harvest or planting season, the agricultural productivity of the village would be severely impaired.[21] For this reason, guinea worm infection is sometimes known as the "empty granary" disease.[21] These losses have been quantified in several regions of West Africa.[22] Therefore, the economic impact of guinea worm infection is almost as serious as its health impact. Moreover, in children, guinea worm infection is also associated with malnutrition and school absenteeism,[22] so that, like the STH infections and schistosomiasis, guinea worm has a major educational impact as well.

There is no straightforward cure for dracunculiasis. Even today, a major approach to treating guinea worm is to use the ancient practice of slowly extracting the worm onto a small stick and then twisting the stick a bit each day. It is believed that the sign of the caduceus, the universal symbol of medicine depicting a snake wrapped around a staff, probably evolved from what was undoubtedly one of the first treatments ever for an infectious disease! Unfortunately, no anthelmintic drug is effective against guinea worm.

The successes in guinea worm control over the past 20 years represent one of the more interesting stories in the field of the NTDs.[23] During the early 1980s, there was great excitement about disease eradication following the successful eradication of smallpox through widespread vaccination. The last naturally occurring case of smallpox was recorded in Somalia in 1977, and the world was certified free of smallpox in 1981. Although there is no vaccine for guinea worm infection, the CDC suggested dracunculiasis as a potential new target for eradication because of its relatively low prevalence compared to that of other helminth infections such as hookworm infection and schistosomiasis. Additional reasons were the observations that guinea worm infection could be prevented by health education and straightforward behavioral changes, such as filtering water through cloth to remove copepods and avoiding public water supplies during active infection. Proof of concept that such measures were effective included previously successful eradication efforts in Uzbekistan, Iran, and in some states of India, such as Tamil Nadu and Gujarat.[24] In 1986, two landmark events occurred. First, the 39th WHA adopted a resolution to eliminate dracunculiasis, and second, former U.S. President Jimmy Carter, together with Dr. Donald Hopkins, began to champion efforts to eradicate the guinea worm. His advocacy began in Pakistan, where he persuaded General Mohammad Zia ul-Haq to step up eradication efforts, and then subsequently in sub-Saharan Africa, where he worked with the leaders of Ghana, Mali, and Nigeria to embark on national control programs. In 1993 Pakistan became the first country to eradicate guinea worm, and by 1995–1996, guinea worm eradication efforts were under way in every country where dracunculiasis was endemic. These efforts were then linked with a new WHA resolution (WHA 50.35), which urged all "Member States, international and nongovernmental organizations and appropriate entities to continue to ensure political support and the availability of much-needed resources for completion of eradication of dracunculiasis as quickly as technically feasible and for the International Commission for the Certification of Dracunculiasis Eradication and its work."[25] The three major elements of these proposed eradication efforts included (i) provision of safe water through the construction of wells (as a source of water free from copepods), filtering of water, and application of larvicidal agents (primarily the agent Temephos [Abate; American Cyanamid]) that destroy copepods; (ii) health education; and (iii) case containment and management.[23] Among the important new tools in this effort was a new and more efficient nylon cloth filter that was developed by DuPont specifically for guinea worm filtration.[23]

Over the last 20 years, the Dracunculiasis Eradication Program (DEP, presently under the direction of Ernesto Ruiz-Tiben) has been an unqualified success. Only 25,000 or so cases of guinea worm infection remain on the planet, of which approximately 80% are in Sudan, where a long-standing civil war has thwarted public health interventions over the last 20 years, and in northern Ghana.[26] Even during the worst years of fighting in war-torn Sudan, former President Carter made surprising gains in fighting guinea worm. In 1995, he negotiated a 4-month-long "Guinea Worm Cease-Fire," with the Carter Center facilitating coordination of eradication activities from both sides, using offices in both Khartoum (the Sudanese capital) and Nairobi.[27] The cease-fire demonstrated that it was possible to continue public health interventions in areas of conflict (in chapter 7, we will see how wars in Angola, the Democratic Republic of the Congo, and Sudan enabled the recrudescence of human African trypanosomiasis).

The control of LF and guinea worm infection, like so many NTD control programs, represents extremely low-cost and cost-efficient measures. For LF, both ivermectin and albendazole are donated free of charge, while DEC is produced generically and can be purchased for just a few pennies per dose. Therefore, LF mass drug administration can be provided for less than US$1 per person (http://www.filariasis.org). Similarly, the estimated cost of the DEP between 1987 and 1998 was $87.5 million or approximately US$5 to $8 per prevented case.[28] In 2000, the Gates Foundation provided another US$28.5 million to continue these activities. The Carter Center is working furiously to ensure that it meets a 2009 target for guinea worm eradication. If the center is successful, it will have been accomplished for well under US$200 million.

In their own ways, LF mass drug administration and the DEP have been wildly successful. The target year for the global eradication of guinea worm is 2009, and given dramatic rates of guinea worm reduction over the last 20 years and now the stepped-up measures in Sudan through a new Sudan Guinea Worm Eradication Program,[29] there is optimism on achieving these goals. Major reasons for success include the availability of simple interventions together with President Carter's high-level advocacy and excellent coordination by the Carter Center and its partners. For LF, wherever elimination efforts have been aggressively pursued, the outcome has been extremely favorable. However, because the magnitude of the LF elimination problem is so much greater than the problem forcing the DEP, the WHO and other organizations estimate that only about one-third or fewer of the 1 billion people at risk for infection have so far received mass drug administration of either DEC or ivermectin. Therefore, we could be looking at many decades before LF elimination is under way in most of the developing world, especially in Africa. Later (in chapter 10), we will see how linking LF control with other NTD mass drug administration programs might soon catalyze greater efficiencies and increase coverage.

Summary Points: LF and Guinea Worm

LF

- LF occurs in an estimated 120 million people in the world's poorest countries, where approximately 1 billion people are at risk for acquiring the infection. Most of the world's cases occur in India and in sub-Saharan Africa, with Southeast Asia, the Pacific, and some tropical regions of the Americas (especially Haiti and northeastern Brazil) accounting for the remainder.
- Approximately 90% of the world's LF cases are caused by the nematode parasite *W. bancrofti*. The adult worms live for 8 years in the lymphatics. They produce microfilariae that enter the bloodstream and are transmitted person to person through a mosquito vector.
- The morbidity and pathology of LF result from adult *W. bancrofti* worms in the lymphatics, which cause dilation (lymphangiectasia), obstruction, lymphedema, and, in some cases, elephantiasis.
- The chronic morbidity and disfigurement resulting from LF exact a huge economic toll, almost $1 billion in losses annually to the Indian economy. Much of this loss is from reduced worker productivity. In addition, the stigma of LF has an enormous but still poorly quantified social impact.
- Transmission of LF in poor rural communities can be interrupted by mass drug administration of anthelmintic drugs that target the microfilariae. These drugs include DEC and ivermectin. Widespread use of DEC in national programs has resulted in the elimination or near elimination of LF in Brazil, China, Egypt, Japan, and Taiwan. In some cases, it has been brought about through use of DEC-fortified salt.
- Despite years of administering DEC or ivermectin, only 21 to 38% coverage of people at risk worldwide has been achieved. Greater efficiencies in coverage might be achieved through integrated NTD control. A WHA resolution has called for the elimination of LF by the year 2020.

Guinea worm

- Dracunculiasis is caused by the guinea worm, *D. medinensis*. Prior to global eradication efforts that began 20 years ago, an estimated 3.5 million people were infected, primarily in Africa and the Middle East and on the Indian subcontinent.
- The adult *D. medinensis* worm grows to almost 1 yard in length and lives in the subcutaneous tissues of the legs and feet (as well as elsewhere). The adult female worm produces a blister that ruptures in water, with the release of immature *D. medinensis* larvae. The larvae are ingested by copepods. Human infection occurs after ingestion of the copepods.

Summary Points *(continued)*

- Stepped-up measures for guinea worm control began in 1986, with former President Carter and the Carter Center spearheading many of the initiatives. The major tools of the DEP include provision of safe water, health education, and case containment. In 1993, Pakistan became the first country to eradicate guinea worm infection.

- Today, only about 25,000 cases of guinea worm infection remain, mostly in Sudan and, to some extent, Ghana. There is optimism that the guinea worm will be eradicated by 2009.

The Blinding Neglected Tropical Diseases: Onchocerciasis (River Blindness) and Trachoma

*I remember vividly those days in what was then called Upper Volta and is now Burkina Faso ...
We had heard, before and during the visit, about the terrible disease called river blindness, and
some had suggested that the World Bank should play a role in doing something about it. We
could hardly pronounce the name of the disease, much less spell onchocerciasis, but were hor-
rified by what we heard about it. Literally millions of people were at risk of a fate that could be
worse than death in that society and time.*

ROBERT MCNAMARA[1]

An estimated 259 million people in the world suffer from visual impairment, and 42 million people are blind.[2] Sadly, 80% of the world's blind people live in developing countries, and the majority (about two-thirds) of the cases of blindness are either preventable or curable.[3] A startling example of how blindness disproportionately affects vulnerable and impoverished people in developing countries is a recent analysis of visual loss in postconflict southern Sudan.[4] Between 1983 and 2005, the second Sudanese civil war killed an estimated 1.9 million civilians, one of the highest death tolls since World War II, and forced the relocation of another 4 million people.[4] Because of its strategic location near oil fields, the Mankien district of Sudan was particularly affected by the conflict (Color Plate 8).[4] A team from Cambridge University found that 4% of the people in postconflict Mankien villages were blind and that almost double that number had poor vision. Therefore, people living under the harsh conditions of postconflict Sudan are six to seven times more likely to become blind than are those living in the rest of the world. The WHO considers blindness a severe public health problem in a community when the local prevalence is 1% or greater;[5] this region of Sudan exceeds even this level by fourfold. Blindness in such resource-poor settings is especially onerous because of the absence of support services found in the industrialized world. Not surprisingly, blind people who live in the settings of rural poverty are at much higher risk of death and injury, possibly as much as fivefold.[6]

Here we will consider the impact of blindness that results from two neglected tropical diseases (NTDs) that are entirely preventable with simple, safe, and effective preventive chemotherapy. Trachoma is a bacterial infection occurring in approximately 84 million persons living in the developing regions of Africa, the Middle East, Central Asia, India, and Southeast Asia. Onchocerciasis is a parasitic helminth infection occurring in an estimated 37 million people, primarily in West and Central Africa.

Onchocerciasis

Onchocerciasis is also known as river blindness because the *Simulium* blackflies that transmit this filarial infection breed along fast-flowing streams. The infection is caused by *Onchocerca volvulus*, a filarial worm with similarities to the parasites causing lymphatic filariasis (LF) and dracunculiasis (chapter 4). The *Onchocerca* adult worms resemble long pieces of pasta up to 20 in. in length, which coil up in fibrous nodules that form under the skin. Both the adult female *Wuchereria bancrofti* worms that cause LF and the adult female *O. volvulus* worms also produce microscopic microfilariae. However, unlike the *W. bancrofti* microfilariae, the *Onchocerca* microfilariae do not enter the bloodstream in large numbers. Instead, they mostly migrate in the skin, where they cause intense itching and disfigurement. However, from the skin some of the microfilariae also reach the eye, where they form small opacities. Over a period of years, sometimes decades, these opacities begin to coalesce and eventually block out light. This progression is the basis by which *O. volvulus* causes blindness in approximately 270,000 people and visual impairment in 500,000.[7–9] Although onchocerciasis is best known as a cause of eye disease and blindness, the manifestations that result from the presence of microfilariae in the skin are almost as severe. These cutaneous manifestations are both highly disfiguring and stigmatizing, and the associated itching has been alleged to be so intense that it can even prompt suicide.

The vast majority of the estimated 37 million infected with onchocerciasis are impoverished subsistence farmers and their families living in West, Central, and parts of East Africa (Color Plate 9). The disease is widely distributed in these regions, where it takes two major forms, a savanna form that is primarily associated with blindness, and a forest form in which skin disease is a more prominent feature.[9] In some savanna communities, there is hyperendemic transmission of onchocerciasis and blindness can be found in 10% or more of poor rural villages, while in the forest zone of West Africa, severe *Onchocerca* skin disease (OSD) afflicts millions of people. In the tropical regions of the Americas, another 140,000 infections occur in Guatemala and the neighboring Chiapas State of Mexico, along the Venezuela-Brazil border, in parts of northern Venezuela along the Caribbean coast and in Ecuador and Colombia.[7,9] Today, new cases of blindness caused by onchocerciasis seldom occur in the Americas, although skin disease is common. Outside Africa and the Americas, a focus of onchocerciasis occurs in Yemen, where the major manifestation is a disfiguring condition of the skin known as sowda.

Humans become infected with onchocerciasis when *Simulium* blackflies, which breed along rivers or streams, deposit *O. volvulus* larvae while biting and feeding on blood (Fig. 5.1).[9] Thus, whereas hookworm infective larvae enter human skin from the soil, both *O. volvulus* and *W. bancrofti* infective larvae gain entry into humans during the bite of an insect vector, a mosquito in the case of *W. bancrofti* and a blackfly for *O. volvulus*. Over the course of approximately 1 year, the larvae then migrate to different areas under the skin of the body (subcutaneous tissues) and develop into adult worms. The fibrous

Figure 5.1 Life cycle of *O. volvulus* (Public Health Image Library, CDC [http://phil.cdc.gov]).

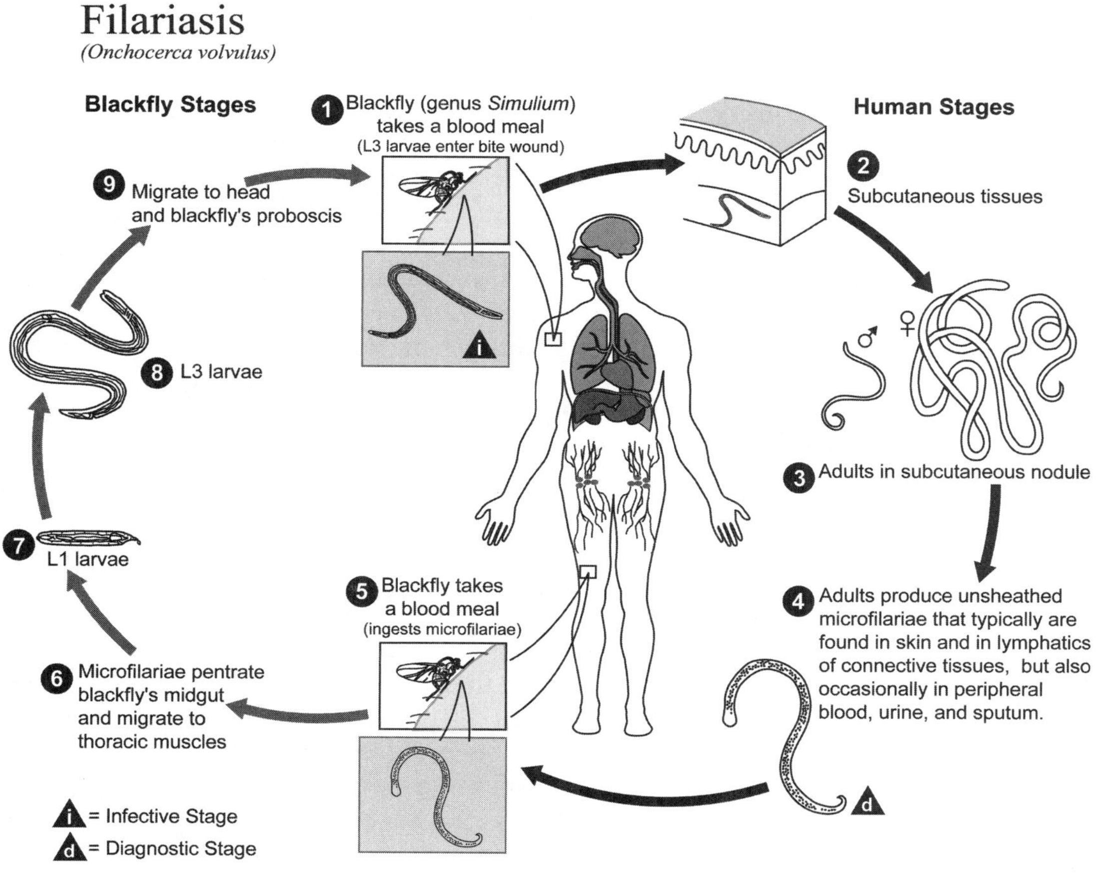

Filariasis
(Onchocerca volvulus)

Blackfly Stages

❶ Blackfly (genus *Simulium*) takes a blood meal
(L3 larvae enter bite wound)

❾ Migrate to head and blackfly's proboscis

❽ L3 larvae

❼ L1 larvae

❻ Microfilariae pentrate blackfly's midgut and migrate to thoracic muscles

❺ Blackfly takes a blood meal
(ingests microfilariae)

Human Stages

❷ Subcutaneous tissues

❸ Adults in subcutaneous nodule

❹ Adults produce unsheathed microfilariae that typically are found in skin and in lymphatics of connective tissues, but also occasionally in peripheral blood, urine, and sputum.

🔺**i** = Infective Stage
🔺**d** = Diagnostic Stage

nodules created by the adult worms lie under the skin, typically located near bony prominences, especially the hip. Encased in these nodules, the adult worms can live for a decade or more.[9,10]

Like *W. bancrofti* and *Dracunculus medinensis*, adult female *O. volvulus* worms grow to enormous lengths, up to 20 in. or more. After fertilization the female worm produces millions of microfilariae (about 500 to 1,500 micro-filariae per day), which then migrate out of the nodules and travel in the skin over all aspects of the body. In some regions of Africa where river blindness is endemic, the density of microfilariae in the skin can be enormous. Some esti-mates suggest that a human can harbor as many as 100 million microfilariae, with some regions of the skin having as many as 2,000 microfilariae per mg of skin.[10] A few of these microfilariae travel to the eye after spreading directly from the adjacent skin. The microfilariae residing in the skin and subcutaneous tissues develop further when they are taken up by blackflies as the insects are feeding on blood. Onchocerciasis is then transmitted to another person when the microfilariae develop into infective larvae (a period of about 6 to 12 days) and are deposited on the skin during a subsequent insect bite.

Onchocerciasis is a debilitating and disabling disease because of resulting disfigurement and blindness. Disfigurement results primarily from OSD, an inflammatory condition that develops in response to the enormous numbers of microfilariae in the skin. In West Africa, OSD is sometimes known locally as craw craw. Contributing to the severity of OSD is the fact that the micro-filariae themselves contain bacterial organisms (of the genus *Wolbachia*). The bacteria are in a sense parasites of the *Onchocerca* parasites and are referred to as endosymbionts. It is thought that as microfilariae die in the skin the released endosymbiotic bacteria serve to incite additional host inflamma-tory responses.[11] Later (in chapter 11) we will see how the *Wolbachia* bacte-rial endosymbionts may be targeted as a novel therapeutic approach for the treatment of onchocerciasis.[11] Most commonly, OSD occurs on the legs, but it is not at all unusual for the entire body to be involved. Over a period of years, the chronic inflammatory reactions in the skin cause it to lose its elasticity and firmness so that the skin takes on a loose and aged appearance.[10] When OSD occurs in the groin, the skin often hangs down in folds, a condition sometimes known as "hanging groin."[7,10] Loss of skin pigmentation also results and can occur in patches, imparting a leopard-like appearance.[10] Simultaneously, mul-tiple nodules under the skin (commonly along the bony prominences of the hip, although hip nodules are more common in Africa than in the Americas) arise because of the presence of adult worms.[10] In Africa's rain forest belt, OSD can be found in 50% or more of the villages.[9,12] In these regions, the stigma surrounding OSD is huge, and it is associated with severe ostracism and psy-chosocial aspects.[13] For instance, in eastern Nigeria, OSD is sometimes known by a nickname that translates as "that which prevents a woman from getting married," and the mistaken belief that this condition results from poor hygiene leads to even further isolation and even reduction in infant breast-feeding.[13,14] Affected men have diminished economic prospects from farming and other rural occupations.[13,14]

Onchocerca eye disease also results from the presence of microfilariae in the skin. Each time a microfilaria enters the eye and dies, it combines with cells from the human immune system to form tiny opacities in the cornea. Over a period of years, sometimes decades, these opacities merge and scar to the point where they block out light. In addition, the major nerve that connects the eye with the brain, the optic nerve, becomes affected, exacerbating the processes leading to blindness.[10] In a typical West or Central African community affected by onchocerciasis, blindness commonly begins to occur in the 4th decade of life and then continues to increase. Thus, in the hardest-hit African communities, individuals who ordinarily are parents and heads of households, typically the family breadwinner, are now rendered blind. Frequently, they are led about their village by their child or grandchild and therefore no longer contribute appreciably to the economic well-being of their farming communities. The economic consequences of this scenario are devastating. When village blindness reaches epidemic proportions, there are too few people who can tend the fields, resulting in food shortages and the abandonment of homelands in otherwise fertile river valleys.[13] When subsistence farmers are forced to migrate into highland regions with poor soils, an entire village can be thrown into poverty.[13] Today in sub-Saharan Africa, we can still find rural savanna villages where 10% or more of the adult population is blind from ochocerciasis.[9]

In the foyer of the World Bank headquarters in Washington, DC, stands a remarkable bronze statue of a child leading a man blinded by onchocerciasis, presumably his father or grandfather, by a stick (Fig. 5.2). Throughout history in sub-Saharan Africa, this tragic scene has been replayed millions of times. To understand the World Bank-onchocerciasis connection, we need to turn the clock back to 1972, when then World Bank President Robert McNamara witnessed firsthand the devastation wrought by onchocerciasis in West Africa. Although he is better known for escalating the Vietnam War as secretary of defense in the Johnson administration, it is not widely appreciated that McNamara also helped to launch one of the world's most successful health and humanitarian programs.[15,16]

Today, the impact of his early efforts to improve the health of the world's poorest people is still widely felt. In 1972, while touring drought-stricken regions of Burkina Faso (then called Upper Volta) in West Africa, McNamara and his wife were overcome by the sight of villages affected by river blindness, particularly the large numbers of middle-aged men and women led by sticks.[15] In the 1970s, it was estimated that more than 60% of some savanna populations were infected with *O. volvulus*, with approximately one-half of the males over the age of 40 years blind.[13] While visiting the capital, Ouagadougou, he met with scientists from ORSTROM (Office de Recherche Scientifique et Technique Outre-Mer), a scientific arm of the French overseas development agency, who informed McNamara that if blackflies could be controlled for as long as adult *O. volvulus* worms live in the human body (10 to 20 years), then in theory transmission of the disease could be interrupted. In response, McNamara held a summit in Paris, which ultimately led to the establishment of the Onchocerciasis Control Program (OCP), a unique partnership of the World Bank, with

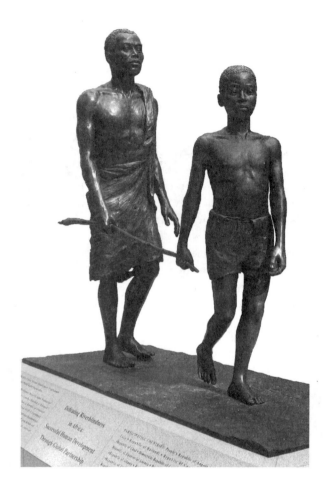

Figure 5.2 A bronze study of a blind man led by a young boy (R. T. Wallen). Reproductions of this statue are located at the World Bank and at the World Health Organization. Photo by Julie Ost.

the World Health Organization, the Food and Agriculture Organization (FAO), and the UN Development Programme (UNDP).[15,16]

Launched in 1974, the OCP followed on the heels of earlier attempts to control populations of the blackfly vector in Ghana and in Francophone West Africa (including Burkina Faso, Ivory Coast, and Mali) led by ORSTROM and other organizations.[16] During its first 14 years of existence, the major focus of the OCP was to interrupt transmission of onchocerciasis by controlling the *Simulium* insect vector. Blackfly populations were controlled by frequent and periodic use of Temephos, an organophosphorus insecticide that destroys *Simulium* larvae. Earlier (in chapter 4) we saw how Temephos was applied to water in order to destroy copepod larvae for the control of guinea worm infection. For onchocerciasis, Temephos was delivered either through aerial spraying (helicopters or fixed-wing aircraft) or by ground application. The rationale for aerial spraying was to reduce blackfly populations in order to stop transmission and then sustain zero transmission for 2 decades or more, a time equivalent to the life of *O. volvulus* in human tissues.[13] Ultimately, the OCP used more environmentally friendly larvicides, often rotating them periodically in order to defeat emerging insect resistance. An important component of the OCP was an emphasis on parallel research in order to continually identify new larvicides.[16] This practice is a useful lesson for 21st-century large-scale efforts to control malaria with bed nets and indoor residual spraying—to date, neither the U.S. government's President's Malaria Initiative (PMI) nor the Global Fund to Fight AIDS, Tuberculosis, and Malaria includes operational research as a prominent component of its control efforts.

In its first few years of existence, the OCP concentrated larvicidal spraying in seven West African countries—Benin, Burkina Faso, Cote d'Ivoire, Ghana, Mali, Niger, and Togo—where in many regions more than 60% of village populations were infected, with blindness rates that exceeded 10%. Despite this intense concentration of disease and misery, in most of the regions of these countries where onchocerciasis was endemic, the OCP was successful in eliminating onchocerciasis, meaning that transmission of the disease was reduced to zero.[16] Because blackflies do not respect international borders, an added key component of the OCP was international cooperation among the seven countries.[13] Ultimately, four additional countries—Guinea, Guinea-Bissau, Senegal, and Sierra Leone—were targeted for aerial spraying after OCP scientists discovered that blackflies were traveling up to 600 km away from the major targeted areas.[13] The achievements of the OCP are impressive. By the time it ceased operations in 2002, it was estimated that the OCP had prevented approximately 600,000 cases of blindness, while 18 million children born in the OCP area were freed from risk of river blindness and 25 million hectares of arable land (which could feed 17 million people) were made available.[16] Even today, some 20 to 30 years after larvicidal spraying began, many regions of West Africa remain onchocerciasis free. Moreover, these efforts were extremely cost-effective; some estimates indicate that OCP achieved its goals for less than US$1 per person.[16]

OCP was successful, but not entirely, because of insecticides and their widespread use. Roughly at the halfway mark in the program, a second control tool was introduced, which greatly enhanced the progress of OCP and still provides a basis for onchocerciasis control programs today. During the 1970s, Merck scientists led by William Campbell discovered a new drug with anthelmintic properties. The precursor of ivermectin (later given the trade name Mectizan) originated from a microorganism (*Streptomyces avermitilis*) living in soil samples obtained from a Japanese golf course![17] Unlike human parasites, veterinary parasites represent a rather large commercial market because of their adverse health impact on livestock. What was so amazing about Merck's role in the story of human onchocerciasis was that, after developing ivermectin for veterinary use, the company did not close the door on developing it for a human disease with no commercial value. Instead, Merck, together with the WHO, began a number of clinical trials in regions of Africa and the Americas where onchocerciasis was endemic, which demonstrated that a single dose of ivermectin was both safe and effective in reducing the density of microfilariae living in human tissue.[16,17] In efforts headed by then Merck CEO Roy Vagelos, the company in 1987 worked successfully with William Foege, the Carter Center's executive director, to establish a unique public-private partnership for donating Mectizan free of charge to anyone who needed the drug for as long as it was needed.[16] The Mectizan Donation Program (http://www.mectizan.org) has since 1988 provided an estimated 400 million treatments for onchocerciasis, as well as for LF.[7]

A key to the success of the OCP was providing poor people with onchocerciasis access to Mectizan. Access was accomplished through an innovative use of community-based drug distributors. The early experience with Mectizan in the OCP was that well-trained and expensive mobile health teams would enter villages where onchocerciasis was endemic, only to find that villagers were often away, tending to their fields or hunting.[13] The excellent safety profile of Mectizan, however, meant that it was both safe and practical for the mobile teams to leave the drug in the village and allow community-based workers to administer it on their own.[13] Eventually these steps led to the creation of a network of community drug distributors, today known as CDTI (community-directed treatment with ivermectin), which has since revolutionized access to this essential medicine. At the same time, many nongovernmental developmental organizations (NGDOs) began to coordinate their activities through CDTI. In the future it is likely that CDTI and CDTI-like programs could provide a mechanism for large-scale interventions against several NTDs, as well as for antimalaria measures, vitamin A distribution, and pediatric vaccinations.[13]

Within a few years after CDTI began, it was clear that the OCP was becoming an important success story, but because the OCP did not cover the disease in Central or East Africa (or in the Americas), there was a need for additional partnerships to cover these regions. The African Programme for Onchocerciasis Control (APOC) built on OCP successes to reach 19 additional African countries—Angola, Burundi, Cameroon, the Central African Republic, Chad, the Democratic Republic of the Congo, the Republic of the Congo, Equatorial Guinea, Ethiopia, Gabon, Kenya, Liberia, Malawi, Mozambique, Nigeria, Rwanda, Sudan, Tanzania, and Uganda—with an initial aim to treat 75 million people annually with Mectizan, but ultimately scaling to 90 million treatments annually.[16,18] CDTI is also a cornerstone of APOC, with ivermectin distributed annually in areas where the number of villagers with *Onchocerca* nodules exceeds 20%.[9] Monitoring and evaluation efforts have determined that CDTI has achieved enormous therapeutic successes in the target APOC countries.[13] Through APOC-sponsored CDTI, approximately 40 million people living in 90,000 villages have received treatments from an estimated 300,000 community distributors.[7] This achievement has been highly cost-effective, estimated at US$6.50 per disability-adjusted life year.[13] APOC is headed by a charismatic and highly effective African woman, Uche Amazigo, who manages the program from offices in Ouagadougou, Burkina Faso, the birthplace of onchocerciasis control. Because APOC integrates into Africa's primary health care system, it has become a model for distributing other interventions. Particularly exciting is the recent observation that CDTI greatly enhances the efficiency of other health interventions. For example, a study conducted by Frank O. Richards of the Carter Center has shown that by piggybacking onto CDTI, antimalaria bed net distribution increased ninefold.[19] As a result, several NGDOs, including the Carter Center and Helen Keller International, are now linking CDTI with malaria control initiatives.[13] Later (in chapter 10), we will see how this is just the beginning of an effort to link multiple NTD and malaria control efforts. In the Americas, the Onchocerciasis Elimination Program for the Americas (OEPA) is focused primarily on the highest-risk countries of the Americas, e.g., Mexico, Guatemala, and Venezuela.[8]

APOC was initially launched as a 12-year program, but it has since been extended until 2010. By that time it is projected that approximately 150 million people will have been protected in 30 countries.[13] However, based on the premise that annual treatments would need to be continued for as long as the adult *O. volvulus* parasites live in the body, it is widely accepted that the activities of APOC or an equivalent program will likely need to be sustained for much longer in order to make a significant impact on the African elimination of onchocerciasis.[7,18] Although this contingency could mean another 20 years of ivermectin coverage, it is unclear whether international funding support for APOC will continue. Later (in chapter 10), we will discuss the possibility of sustaining support of APOC through an expansion of its mandate to include other NTD control measures.

A new challenge to global efforts to control onchocerciasis is the observation that *O. volvulus* resistance to ivermectin may have developed in some specific regions of Ghana and possibly other OCP countries.[20] Presumably this resistance was brought about by repeated mass drug administration of Mectizan over a period of 19 years. At this time it is unclear whether the diminished efficiencies of ivermectin in Ghana are truly a result of resistance and/or whether resistance will become widespread as it did for chloroquine, the antimalarial, or whether ivermectin resistance is a self-contained problem that will not affect long-term control. Without the benefit of having additional backup drugs in hand, we have no choice but to continue to aggressively pursue CDTI in most of the regions where onchocerciasis is endemic. Identification of possible emerging drug resistance to ivermectin, however, points out the need for constant vigilance in developing and testing new control tools, which could include new drug development. Later (in chapter 11), we will examine the prospects of new anthelmintic drugs for onchocerciasis, which are based on targeting the parasite's *Wolbachia* bacterial endosymbionts, and even the possibility that an anti-*Onchocerca* vaccine could be developed.

Trachoma

Trachoma is an infection caused by the bacterium *Chlamydia trachomitis* affecting approximately 84 million people and causing blindness in 5 to 6 million people. It is the most important cause of infectious blindness worldwide, accounting for approximately 15% of all of the world's cases of blindness.[21] Like the other NTDs, trachoma is an infection that occurs only in the poorest people of the world. The infection is spread from person to person on dirty hands and clothing, but it is also carried by flies, which can carry the *Chlamydia* bacteria from the eye discharges of one person to another. For that reason, the disease often strikes entire families. Moreover, women are affected three times more than men. According to the nonprofit International Trachoma Initiative (ITI) (http://www.trachoma.org), based in New York City, when a woman who runs the household can no longer work, the burden falls on the daughter, who is forced to leave school, in turn losing her opportunity for education. Such an impact on women and the close association between trachoma and filth and flies ensure a tight link between the disease and poverty. Therefore, trachoma, like onchocerciasis, is an excellent example of an NTD that not only occurs in the setting of poverty but helps to promote it as well. An estimated US$5.3 billion is lost annually from the global trachoma disease burden.[22]

At the turn of the 20th century, trachoma was a major reason why poor European immigrants were prevented from entering the United States. Back then, it was a common practice for U.S. Public Health Service physicians assigned to Ellis Island to screen potential immigrants by turning up their eyelids and looking for signs of the disease. During the early part of the 20th century, trachoma was a common disease in the United States, particularly on Indian reservations, where crowding, poverty, and lack of clean water combined to create conditions favorable for transmission.[23] In 1913, President Woodrow Wilson signed antitrachoma legislation making the control of this infection a priority for the United States. As a result of improved housing and standards of living, trachoma is no longer a major public health threat,[23] although the infection still occurs sporadically among the Navajo and other Native American tribes in the West.[24] Today, the disease principally occurs throughout the poorest developing countries of Africa, Central Asia, the Middle East, India, and Southeast Asia (Color Plate 10). Trachoma is also found in a few regions of the Americas (Mexico and and Brazil) and the Pacific region, including Australian regions that are home to aboriginal populations.

Unlike many NTDs discussed previously, which depend on adequate moisture and rainfall to ensure survival of parasite larval stages in the soil, in water, or in arthropod vectors, trachoma more often occurs in dry and dusty environments, particularly those without adequate sanitation and with large populations of flies. The environmental risk factors of dryness and filth for trachoma have been summarized by the six Ds (dryness, dust, dirt, dung, discharge, and density [overcrowding]) or the five Fs (flies, feces, faces, fingers, and fomites).[21] Dirty and unwashed faces, as well as human or animal feces on the ground, attract flies that spread the disease.[21] Other important risk factors include lack of adequate access to clean water, which requires villagers to walk long distances for their water supply. This task in turn lessens the likelihood of adequate hygiene.[21] The absence of education, especially maternal education, is another risk factor.[22]

Trachoma is a chronic infection that usually begins in childhood, sometimes with redness (pinkeye), itching, and pain[21,25] (Fig. 5.3). The disease and blindness result from recurrent and multiple infections with *C. trachomitis*,

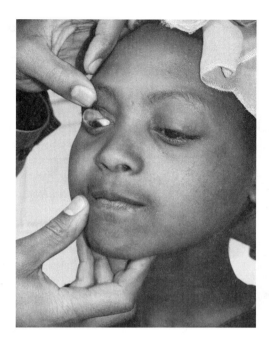

Figure 5.3 Trachoma patient—a fifth-grade student—in Silti Zone, Ethiopia. (©International Trachoma Initiative; photo by Beth D. Weinstein.)

which occur over a period of 10 to 20 years. During this time, recurrent infection leads to scarring of the eyelids. When the scarred eyelids turn inward, the lashes scratch the surface of the eyeball, leading to inflammation and scarring of the cornea (an ordinarily transparent part of the eye) and ultimately blindness. These later stages are known as trichiasis.[25]

Because these pathologic processes are insidious and occur over a period of years or even decades, and because they occur only among poor people usually in remote areas, trachoma has often been overlooked as a serious public health problem. Adding to the neglect of trachoma is the commonness of this condition in areas made inaccessible by conflict or postconflict turmoil. However, over the last several years, the WHO, together with the ITI, has developed an innovative strategy of trachoma management and prevention that goes by the acronym SAFE:[21,26]

- S is for simple surgery, for the relief of trichiasis to prevent corneal scarring. In many countries health professionals other than physicians, such as nurses and specialized ophthalmic assistants, can be trained to perform this simple operation, which involves making a slit in the eyelid and peeling back a portion to prevent further scarring.
- A is for antibiotics. The major antibiotic used is a single oral dose of azithromycin, marketed by Pfizer as the drug Zithromax. Zithromax has largely replaced tetracycline, which had to be administered topically for a period of 4 to 6 weeks.
- F is for facial hygiene. Children with clean faces have a reduced likelihood of developing severe trachoma, especially when face washing is combined

with administration of Zithromax. Face washing can also help to interrupt transmission.

- E is for environmental improvement. This component relies on improving access to clean water and improving sanitation and latrines to reduce fly populations. Combined with health education, environmental change is critical for reducing transmission.

One of the most important breakthroughs in the global control of trachoma was the discovery that a single dose of azithromycin was as effective as 4 to 6 weeks of topical tetracycline for the treatment of trachoma.[26] Azithromycin bears some structural resemblance to tetracycline, but its chemistry is modified so that it achieves greater penetration inside human cells. Since *C. trachomitis* lives inside cells (it is an intracellular bacterium), this finding afforded an opportunity to achieve similar antibiotic efficacy with fewer doses. Although Zithromax was developed primarily as the Z-PAK for the treatment of outpatients with pneumonia and other community-acquired infections, during the 1990s, Pfizer, together with the Edna and McConnell Clark Foundation, conducted clinical trials showing that a single dose of the drug was also effective for treating trachoma. In 1998 Pfizer and the Clark Foundation established the ITI, which included Pfizer's donation of US$60 million worth of azithromycin.[26] Since Zithromax was one of Pfizer's best-selling products and since there was a risk that the donated drug would be sold in developing countries on the black market,[26] the donation of this product is considered an extraordinary gesture of corporate philanthropy and one that rivals Merck's Mectizan Donation Program. Formerly under the leadership of Joe Cook and Jacob Kumaresan, ITI is presently headed by its president, Ibrahim Jabr.

Through the activities of ITI as well as of other organizations dedicated to fighting blindness, such as Helen Keller International, the WHO has established guidelines to administer azithromycin en masse in affected communities where the prevalence of trachomatous folliculitis exceeds 20%. In some cases, mass drug administration is used when the prevalence exceeds 5%, although targeted treatment of specific groups is sometimes warranted in these settings.[27] In 1999, Morocco became the first country to embark on a comprehensive program of trachoma control, which used both the SAFE strategy and single-dose azithromycin.[26] Before the control campaign, an estimated 5.4% of the population was affected, with all of the cases in five southeastern rural provinces.[26] To ensure success, Morocco's National Blindness Control Program created a comprehensive partnership comprised of five government ministries including health and education; international organizations such as ITI, Helen Keller, UNICEF, and WHO; bilateral and multilateral agencies; and local nongovernmental organizations.[26] Their efforts included mobile surgical units staffed by physicians and nurses to perform surgery, administer Zithromax, provide health education, and construct new latrines and wells.[26] In 2005, Morocco became the first developing country to successfully interrupt the transmission of trachoma through the SAFE strategy and to seek certification that it had eliminated the disease. In November 2006, the king of Morocco hosted a high-profile celebration to mark the end of mass distribution of antibiotics.[26] The ITI is currently supporting trachoma control programs in 11 other countries, including nine African nations (Tanzania, Ghana, Niger, Mali, Ethiopia, Kenya, Sudan, Mauritania, and Senegal) and two Asian ones (Nepal and Vietnam).[26,27] In Ghana, Mali, and Niger, ITI has successfully integrated treatments for trachoma with other NTD control measures. In all, approximately one-half of the populations of Mali and Niger were treated in 2007.

Summary Points: the Blinding NTDs

Blindness

- Eighty percent of the world's blind people live in developing countries.
- The majority of the cases of blindness are either preventable or curable.

Onchocerciasis

- Onchocerciasis is also known as river blindness because the *Simulium* blackflies that transmit this filarial infection breed along fast-flowing streams.
- The infection is caused by *O. volvulus*, a filarial worm with similarities to the parasites causing LF and dracunculiasis.
- An estimated 37 million people are infected with onchocerciasis, which is responsible for blindness in approximately 270,000 people and visual impairment in another 500,000.
- Onchocerciasis also produces a serious, debilitating, and stigmatizing skin disease (OSD).
- The OCP was launched in 1974 following the advocacy of then World Bank President Robert McNamara. Over the next 30 years, OCP helped to facilitate the elimination of onchocerciasis in large regions of 11 West African countries.
- The cornerstone of OCP was initially insecticidal spraying, but it was gradually replaced by annual treatments with ivermectin. Since 1988, ivermectin has been donated by Merck through its Mectizan Donation Program.
- Today, onchocerciasis control continues through the activities of the APOC and the OEPA. The cornerstone of APOC is CDTI.
- The future of onchocerciasis control is uncertain, pending the unresolved future funding for APOC, the role of integrated NTD control, and the specter of ivermectin resistance.

Trachoma

- Trachoma is an infection caused by the bacterium *C. trachomitis*; it occurs in approximately 84 million people and causes blindness in 5 to 6 million people.

Summary Points *(continued)*

- It is the most common cause of infectious blindness worldwide, accounting for approximately 15% of all of the world's cases of blindness.
- Trachoma spreads from person to person on dirty hands and clothing. The disease is also carried by flies that can carry the *Chlamydia* bacteria from the eye discharges of one person to another.
- Women are affected three times more than are men.
- An estimated $5.3 billion is lost annually from the global disease burden.
- The environmental risk factors of dryness and filth for trachoma have been summarized by the six Ds (dryness, dust, dirt, dung, discharge, and density [overcrowding]) or the five Fs (flies, feces, faces, fingers, and fomites).
- Trachoma is a chronic infection that usually begins in childhood; blindness results from recurrent and multiple infections occurring over a period of 10 to 20 years.
- An innovative strategy of trachoma management and prevention goes by the acronym SAFE—Surgery, Antibiotics, Face Washing, and Environmental Control.
- A breakthrough in the global control of trachoma was the discovery that a single dose of azithromycin was as effective as 4 to 6 weeks of administering topical tetracycline. Pfizer in association with the ITI is providing large-scale donations of azithromycin (Zithromax) to 13 countries where trachoma is endemic.
- In 2006, Morocco became the first country to eliminate trachoma by using the SAFE strategy and single-dose Zithromax.

chapter 6

The Mycobacterial Infections:
Buruli Ulcer and Leprosy

Witches are known mainly for spreading mysterious diseases in Ghanaian societies, like tuber-culosis, Buruli, and leprosy. In my case, I think it's caused by witchcraft because I have good hygiene. I hope it is only a witch who can bring such a strange sickness or disease to someone because God the Almighty loved us and will not bring us such a sickness.

BURULI PATIENT FROM GHANA[1]

Now the leper on whom the sore is, his clothes shall be torn and his head bare; and he shall cover his mustache, and cry, "Unclean! Unclean!" He shall be unclean. All the days he has the sore he shall be unclean. He is unclean, and he shall dwell alone; his dwelling shall be outside the camp.

LEVITICUS 13[1]

Mycobacteria are slim bacteria with unusual growth requirements and unique structural and biochemical properties that place them in their own category of microbes. Unlike many other types of bacteria, the mycobacteria exhibit the ability to grow inside cells of our immune system known as macrophages. This ability is a remarkable feature because immunologists consider macrophages "professional killer cells," i.e., the cells best armed to ward off invading bacteria and other pathogens. Through evolution, however, the mycobacteria have adapted such that they not only thrive and multiply in macrophages, but in some cases actually use the macrophages as vehicles for transport to specific body tissues.[2]

Tuberculosis (TB), caused by the bacterium *Mycobacterium tuberculosis*, is the best-known mycobacterial infection of humans. As urbanization increased during the 18th and 19th centuries, TB became known as the "white plague" and may have caused up to 30% of all deaths in Europe, including those of some of its leading intellectuals, writers, and composers, such as the Brontë sisters, Chekhov, Chopin, Goethe, Keats, and Rousseau.[2] Today, TB remains one of the great killers of humankind, responsible for an estimated 1.6 million deaths annually, with the largest number of deaths in Africa, followed by Southeast Asia (http://www.theglobalfund.org/en/about/tuberculosis/default/asp). In Africa, TB is a particular crisis because of its high mortality rate in individuals coinfected with HIV/AIDS. TB is now also an important emerging problem in the countries of the former USSR, where a multidrug-resistant form of the infection is becoming widespread.

In response to the enormous global burden of disease from TB, the Group of Eight governments are financing large-scale TB control programs through the Global Fund to Fight AIDS, Tuberculosis, and Malaria. These Global Fund grants are treating an estimated 3 million people through approved therapy known as "DOTS" (originally an acronym used for "direct observed treatment for TB" but now a brand for a multicomponent international TB control strategy).[3] Similarly, more than 22 million patients have been treated through the WHO's Stop TB Partnership. The Stop TB Partnership is a network of international organizations, donors, and countries, as well as governmental and nongovernmental organizations, established in 2000 with the goal of eliminating TB as a public health problem (http://www.stoptb.org). Thus, through high-level advocacy, TB has become a major target for global health activities and philanthropy.

Here we consider two other serious and important mycobacterial infections of the poor—Buruli ulcer and leprosy, which have not benefited from the same level of advocacy as TB. Buruli ulcer and leprosy are two highly disfiguring and stigmatizing NTDs occurring among exclusively among the impoverished living in developing countries.

Buruli ulcer

Buruli ulcer (also known as Buruli disease) is a disfiguring skin infection caused by *Mycobacterium ulcerans*. The name of this condition comes from a region located near the Nile River in Uganda where large numbers of cases were reported in 1962;[4] however, earlier descriptions can be traced as far back as 1897, to those by Sir Albert Cook, a British medical missionary.[5] The identification of a mycobacterium as the cause of ulcers in Buruli disease patients was reported in 1948.[5,6] Today Buruli ulcer occurs primarily in tropical and humid regions of West Africa, where since 1980 large numbers of cases have been reported from Benin, Cote d'Ivoire, and Ghana (Color Plate 11).[5,6] Some investigators believe that the number of cases of Buruli disease in West Africa has increased since 1980, possibly because of deforestation and other environmental factors.[6] In other parts of sub-Saharan Africa, too, the disease is endemic, and it has been reported in some countries outside Africa, including Australia, where aboriginal populations are particularly vulnerable. After tuberculosis, Buruli ulcer is probably the second or third most common myco-bacterial infection of humans, although because the disease occurs primarily in remote areas of the tropics, we lack good global disease burden estimates.

Color Plate 12 shows the terrible ulceration and destruction that can result from *M. ulcerans* infection. Buruli ulcer strikes primarily school-age children. Typically, the ulcer begins as a small painless nodule immediately under the skin, but this nodule subsequently breaks down into a large ulcer.[6] The ulcers usually appear on the limbs but can occur almost anywhere, including the face, breast, and genitals.[6] It is believed that the *M. ulcerans* bacteria that cause Buruli create the ulcers by producing a unique chemical toxin that is destructive to the skin and underlying subcutaneous tissue. A fair amount of scientific informa-tion is known about the so-called mycolactone toxin of the Buruli bacterium, including its size, chemical composition, and the biochemical mechanisms by which it destroys human skin.[7] The entire genome of *M. ulcerans* has recently been sequenced, with the finding that the genes encoding the enzymes needed to produce the mycolactone exist on genetic elements known as plasmids,[6,8] i.e., circular molecules of DNA that exist and replicate separately from chro-mosomal DNA.

Although it is typically painless and rarely results in death, the ulcer of Buruli disease has a number of catastrophic consequences for the patient. For instance, tissue destruction sometimes results in infection of the underlying bone (known as osteomyelitis) or it can necessitate limb amputation. Also, if lesions occur near joints such as the knee or elbow, the subsequent healing can result in contractures that prevent the use of the limb.

The socioeconomic consequences of Buruli ulcer are just as profound. As suggested by the opening quotation of this chapter, there are widespread beliefs that witchcraft and curses play an important role in transmitting the disease.[1] Such beliefs include the concept of the "evil eye," which holds that the Buruli lesion can be made worse when it is seen by certain individuals. A team from Groningen University Hospital in The Netherlands recently studied beliefs about and attitudes toward Buruli ulcer in Ghana.[1] Through patient inter-views, they gained a wealth of information about the stigmatizing and poverty-promoting aspects of the disease. For instance, regarding the concept of the evil eye, the Groningen team obtained this statement about one patient's ulcer:[1]

> If a lot of people see my wound, it might not heal. If all people start to talk about it, stare at it and are surprised by it, it would not heal either.… I always want the door closed during changing of dressings, to protect it from evil eyes.

This statement illustrates how someone afflicted with Buruli ulcer could isolate himself from his community and even medical attention. Among the stigma-tizing aspects of Buruli ulcer, the Groningen team found that even though the disease is not transmitted from person to person, fear of acquiring the disease was a major reason to shun individuals with the condition. Leading to further isolation was the belief that some people with Buruli ulcer are cursed or were victims of witchcraft.[1]

> If the family has a curse or witchcraft, I would think less of the family. I can hear from rumors in the community if the cause of the disease is a curse or witchcraft.

It was further found that young people with Buruli ulcer have diminished prospects for marriage or leadership positions in their villages.[1]

Although Buruli ulcer is certainly not transmitted through witchcraft, the exact transmission mechanism is still under scientific investigation. It has been observed that Buruli ulcer occurs in tropical areas of sub-Saharan Africa where there are either slow-moving rivers or other bodies of water. One exciting finding is the recovery of *M. ulcerans* or *M. ulcerans* DNA from some of the aquatic insects living in regions of endemicity, usually either from their salivary glands or the biofilm on their legs.[9]

This finding has led to the hypothesis that Buruli is either a waterborne infection (swimming in rivers is a risk factor for infection) or a vector-borne infection or possibly some combination of the two.[6] Possibly, children place themselves at risk for acquiring Buruli ulcer when they first begin swimming and are exposed to either insect bites or the *M. ulcerans* microbes on the insect biofilm.[6] So far, however, information on the possible role of insect vectors in the transmission of *M. ulcerans* has not led to new preventive approaches for Buruli ulcer. Moreover, attempting to discourage children from frequent water contact is not a practical solution for large-scale prevention in regions of endemicity, just as it is not a practical solution for the prevention of schistosomiasis, another waterborne NTD.

The management and treatment of Buruli ulcer are a complex and difficult undertaking, especially in the remote tropical regions of West Africa. Although the *M. ulcerans* bacterium is susceptible to a number of antibiotics when this microorganism is cultured in the laboratory and exposed to different concentrations of antibiotics in the test tube (in vitro), it is less clear whether these same antibiotics work well in infected patients. When the ulcers become too large and there is massive tissue destruction, it is thought that insufficient amounts of antibiotics can enter the affected area.[5,6] Therefore, the most effective treatment of large ulcers requires not only access to essential antibiotics such as rifampin and streptomycin (i.e., drugs similar to those used for the treatment of other mycobacterial infections, including TB), but also access to some surgical treatments, such as removal of dead tissue (a process known as debridement), excision of the ulcer, and sometimes skin grafting. Even with surgery, however, there is a high relapse rate for the condition,[5] and sadly, there are very few skilled surgeons or other health care professionals who are both adept at these treatments and prepared to establish surgical practices in the remote areas of tropical West Africa where Buruli ulcer is endemic.

In this sense, Buruli ulcer represents a "perfect storm" of neglect. Like so many other NTDs, it occurs only in remote and rural areas of the tropics, so that we do not even know how many people are actually afflicted by this condition. Moreover, the disfigurement and stigma of Buruli ulcer, because of its alleged links to witchcraft, curses, and the evil eye, cause individuals to be shunned by their communities. Such people are not brought to the attention of the medical services even in the few instances when health care is available. Finally, we have no easy solutions for either treating or preventing this condition, and there is an urgent need for research on Buruli disease in order to identify its mode of transmission as a basis for designing innovative prevention strategies. In response to the disease's profoundly neglected status, the WHO launched the Global Buruli Ulcer Initiative in 1998 in order to coordinate international Buruli control efforts, as well as to establish an international research agenda.[5] These efforts led in 2004 to a World Health Assembly resolution that called for increased surveillance and control and for efforts to intensify research on new approaches to treat and prevent Buruli disease.[5]

One promising modality for preventing Buruli ulcer is the development of a safe and effective vaccine. Based on large-scale efforts to develop a vaccine for TB, including those of the Gates Foundation-supported Aeras Global TB Vaccine Foundation (http://www.aeras.org), several modalities of vaccination that could be applied to potential Buruli vaccines have been developed. These approaches include the development of recombinant vaccines and DNA vaccines.[10] Such vaccines could exploit parallel efforts to mine the *M. ulcerans* genome in order to identify new target antigens. To date, however, no Buruli vaccines are in clinical trials. The hurdles to developing such antipoverty vaccines will be discussed later (in chapter 11) in more detail.

Leprosy

When it comes to stigma, the mycobacterial infection known as leprosy may have it head and shoulders above the other NTDs, at least in its historical record in the "civilized" ancient worlds of Greece and Rome and in medieval Europe.[11,12] Because of its notorious and profoundly disfiguring clinical features, there are several excellent accounts of leprosy in ancient texts, and some scholars believe that leprosy represents the first infectious disease to be accurately described. In ancient Egypt, where some investigators conjecture that leprosy originated, Pharaoh Ramses II (1379–1290? BCE) banished an estimated 80,000 lepers to live on the edge of the Sahara Desert,[11] while Leviticus, the third book of the Pentateuch, records that Moses received specific instructions on how to diagnose lepers and declare them "unclean."[1,11] There are numerous references to "leprosy" in both the Old Testament and the New Testament,[1,12] although it is likely that many of the sores described in these writings were probably other infections having cutaneous manifestations. Possibly more than any other ancient text, the Bible probably articulated in the greatest detail the stigmatizing aspects of an NTD.[1]

While leprosy may have originated in Egypt, some medical historians who have read accounts of diseases resembling leprosy in the ancient Chinese texts and in the Hindu writings of the Veda consider it more likely that leprosy originated in Asia.[12] Possibly, it was introduced into Anatolia (Asia Minor) and later ancient Greece and Rome by ancient trade routes or by the armies of Alexander the Great (356–323 BCE).[11,12] Irwin W. Sherman of the University of California states that Hippocrates (470–380 BCE) never described leprosy because he never saw it.[12] This observation partly reinforces the concept that biblical leprosy might have been a constellation of other infectious and even some non-infectious conditions. According to Sherman and others, some of this confusion arises because the Hebrew word *saraath* was used to describe a variety of skin conditions and was translated into Greek about 300 years before Christ as *lepros*, meaning "scaly."

One of the earliest accurate descriptions of leprosy in Europe is dated 150 CE.[12] Analysis of bones recovered from cemeteries in Europe indicates that the disease became widespread in medieval Europe, where it was sometimes known as leontiasis because of the resemblance between the faces of afflicted patients and lions. During this period specialized homes or hospitals for lepers were established and were known as leprosaria or lazarettos from the biblical sore-infested beggar, Lazarus.[11,12] In medieval Europe, the lazarettos often functioned more as monasteries than as hospitals as we now know them. Lepers were routinely banished to such institutions because of widespread fear of contracting the disease. The medical writer Berton Roueché found that lepraphobia was extant throughout medieval Europe and reached its pinnacle in the 12th, 13th, and 14th centuries.[11] This period coincided with the height of the leprosy epidemic in Europe. Examples of lepraphobia included the requirement that lepers endure their own mock funeral as a prelude to their banishment either to the lazaretto or to a lifetime of begging, with the added requirement that they announce their presence in the community by a self-imposed ringing of a "Lazarus bell."[11] Other lepers were not so lucky and were burned at the stake or buried alive.[11,12] The origins of the leprosy epidemic in medieval Europe are unknown, although it has been suggested that knights returning from the Crusades were a contributing factor.[12] There was even a spiritual order of leprosy-infected knights known as the Order of Lazarus.[12] Following the medieval period, leprosy apparently became much less common. The reasons for this purported decrease are still a subject of speculation, with one major theory arguing that, with the widespread emergence of TB around this time (possibly in part from increasing urbanization), there were large populations of TB-exposed and -infected patients who developed cross-immunity to leprosy.[13] In this way, infection with *M. tuberculosis* functionally may have acted as a partially effective vaccine against *M. leprae* infection.

The United States has also had a long and interesting association with leprosy patients. By the early 20th century, it had been noted that considerable numbers of leprosy patients were living in the continental United States, especially in Louisiana. In testimony given before Congress in 1916, witnesses noted that lepers in the United States were living under horrible conditions.[14] Some 20 years before it was designated as a national leprosarium, the Indian Camp Plantation in Louisiana began housing lepers and treating them with a novel therapy, developed in India, calling for application of chaulmoogra oil. Whether this is an effective treatment remains controversial, although some studies conducted over the past 3 decades find antileprosy effects. The treatment and care of the patients were administered by the Sisters of an order founded by St. Vincent de Paul known as the Daughters of Charity.[14] The National Hansen's Disease Center, as it ultimately became known, lasted for more than 100 years until it finally closed its doors in 1999 (Fig. 6.1). During that time, it was the only inpatient facility for treating leprosy patients in the continental United States. When patients entered Carville, they were frequently abandoned by their families and friends.[14] For the lepers at Carville, the hospital staff and patients became their families, with the hospital and its grounds functioning as a self-contained village containing its own dental office, cafeteria, cemetery, and even a jail.[14] Well into the middle of the 20th century, patients with leprosy were highly discriminated against in the United States, even to the point where they were refused entry to public restrooms or access to public transportation.[15] Chinese-Americans were particularly victimized on the mistaken belief that they were a frequent source of the disease.[12]

An equally extraordinary story of American leprosy is the formation of the Molokai Colony in Hawaii. During the middle of the 19th century, a Hawaiian king ordered lepers to a quarantine area on the island of Molokai. An area surrounded by the Pacific Ocean on three sides and by steep cliffs on the fourth was chosen. Many of those sentenced to Molokai were pushed off ships several

Figure 6.1 National Hansen's Disease Center, Carville, LA (Public Health Image Library, CDC [http://phil.cdc.gov]).

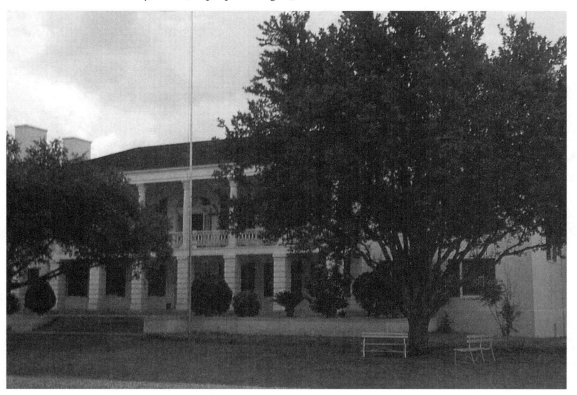

hundred yards from the shore and forced to swim to the island.[12] In the late 1800s, the Honolulu Catholic mission sent Father Damien (Joseph Damien de Veuster), a Belgian Roman Catholic missionary, to Molokai. For more than a decade, Father Damien took care of leprosy patients, before he himself contracted leprosy and died on the island.[12] Known as the "Martyr of Molokai," Father Damien was beatified in 1995 by Pope John Paul II.[12] Today a bronze statue of Father Damien stands in the U.S. Capitol (Fig. 6.2).

Today, as the result of widespread use of a cocktail of antimycobacterial drugs known as MDT (multidrug therapy), the global registered prevalence of leprosy has been reduced to approximately 224,000 cases, with an estimated 259,000 new cases detected annually.[15] Leprosy has therefore been eliminated in all but 10 countries. According to the World Health Organization, leprosy is considered eliminated in a country as a public health problem once the prevalence of the disease diminishes to less than one leprosy case per 10,000 individuals.[15] The highest rates of the infection are currently believed to occur in Central and Southern Africa (Angola, the Central African Republic, the Democratic Republic of the Congo, Madagascar, Mozambique, and

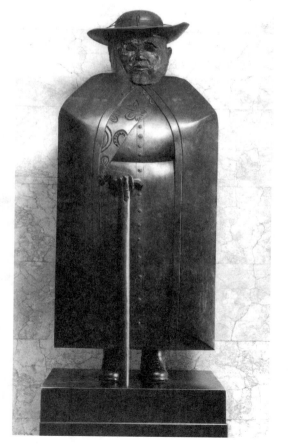

Figure 6.2 Bronze Statue of Father Damien at the U.S. Capitol (http://www.aoc.gov/cc/art/nsh/damien.cfm).

Tanzania), as well as in Brazil, India, and Nepal.[15] Most of these active cases occur in India. Another 2 to 3 million people are considered permanently disabled by leprosy.

Leprosy is caused by *Mycobacterium leprae*. The organism was discovered in the late 1800s by the Norwegian scientist G. H. Armauer Hansen, and the bacterium is one of the first to be implicated as a cause of human disease.[16,17] All mycobacteria, including *M. ulcerans*, *M. tuberculosis*, and *M. leprae*, are known as "acid-fast" organisms because they stain red after specific dyes are used; they are usually seen in clumps or in palisades under the microscope (Color Plate 13). Leprosy is most likely transmitted from the nasal secretions of infected individuals; it has been estimated that a single individual might shed as many as 10 million living leprosy bacilli daily.[16] Exactly how leprosy is subsequently transmitted to another individual is not known, although it is suspected that transmission probably occurs either via the respiratory route or through broken skin.[16] Generally speaking, close contact with a leprosy patient, typically a household member, is required for transmission of leprosy from a patient to a healthy person.[16] Humans are the only major natural host of leprosy, although the infection has also been detected in chimpanzees and other nonhuman primates. Of interest is the finding that the nine-banded armadillo can also support the growth of *M. leprae*.

Not everyone exposed to *M. leprae* develops clinical signs of leprosy.[16] As noted above, the infection is not easily transmitted unless there is very close contact. Even when transmission occurs, a majority of people infected may never show signs or symptoms of the disease. In those who become sick with leprosy, the clinical features usually take up to several years to develop.[16] By the time clinical features are present, large numbers of *M. leprae* microorganisms are usually replicating in the skin and in the peripheral nerves. In the early stages of the disease, peripheral nerve damage results in tingling or absence of sensation. Sometimes burns occur because the patient does not notice exposure to flames or other sources of heat.[16]

Following the initial manifestations of leprosy, the disease usually proceeds along one of two clinical courses.[16] The majority of patients develop the so-called tuberculoid form of the disease. Such patients have the ability to mount strong immunological responses against *M. leprae* microbes and, as a result, develop only localized disease such as loss of sensation or weakness (or both) in the face, hand, leg, foot, or some other body part.[16] Skin lesions resembling plaques also occur on the face, surfaces of the limbs, the back, and the buttocks. Far more severe is the lepromatous form of leprosy. This condition occurs in a much smaller subset of patients who (for reasons that are still not completely elucidated) fail to mount a vigorous immunological response to their *M. leprae* infection.[16] Because replication of the leprosy microorganisms goes unchecked, the bacilli can disseminate widely in the skin and nerves and even invade the eyes, nose, and mouth.[16] Bone invasion can occur, and the testes can also be affected. Massive replication and infiltration of the *M. leprae* bacilli in the skin cause it to become thickened, nodular, and shiny.[16] This condition is accompanied by a deformity of the earlobes and a loss of the eyebrows and eyelashes.[16]

The disfigurement is often worsened by burns and other injuries. Blindness and visual impairments result from destruction in the cornea. Even today there is an enormous stigma from leprosy in developing countries.[17]

An important breakthrough in the global control of leprosy was the development of antimicrobial drugs to treat *M. leprae* infection and a demonstration of their efficacy. One of the first drugs shown to be effective for leprosy treatment was the sulfone compound dapsone. However, because enormous numbers of *M. leprae* mycobacteria live in a patient with lepromatous leprosy, the rate of mutations in the bacterium's genetic material is such that microbial drug resistance was noted early on as a common problem. Drug resistance is also a common problem in patients being treated for TB. During the 1980s, however, the medical community began to circumvent the problem of drug resistance by designing and administering a combination package of several antimycobacterial drugs.[18] Today, the most widely used drug regimen includes dapsone, which is administered together with the antibacterial drugs rifampin (also known as rifampicin) and clofazimine.[18] The regimen requires a full year of treatment, with dapsone and clofazimine administered daily and rifampin once a month.[16]

Within a decade of widespread use of MDT, the World Health Assembly adopted a resolution to eliminate leprosy as a public health problem by the year 2000.[18] Through the generosity of both the Sasakawa Foundation and the drug company Novartis, an estimated 13 to 14 million people have so far received MDT free of charge, and all but 10 of 122 countries where leprosy was once endemic have eliminated leprosy.[18] The barriers to leprosy elimination in the remaining 10 countries (most of the cases occur in Brazil, India, Nepal, Madagascar, Mozambique, and Tanzania) are those in common with many other NTD control and elimination efforts, including the remoteness of many rural areas where these diseases occur and the lack of adequate health care facilities.[18] However, another problem unique to leprosy as compared to most other NTDs is the relatively complicated three-drug regimen that must be used to ensure a patient is adequately treated.[18]

The WHO and other international health agencies are also facing a larger problem of whether their proposed target of reducing prevalence to less than 1 per 10,000 is appropriate and whether it has an adequate scientific rationale. The suggestion has been put forward that the 1-per-10,000 goal is artificial and is more of a political target than a scientific one.[18,19] In addition, several leprosy researchers believe that there are many more cases of leprosy in the world than the ones presently registered by the WHO and that consequently many more individuals should be on MDT but are not.[17,19] In 1999, a new Global Alliance for the Elimination of Leprosy (GAEL) was established in order to make a serious last push for leprosy elimination.[18] Subsequently, an independent evaluation of the GAEL program has recommended changing strategies, with less of a focus on elimination and instead more on creating a new approach that focuses on long-term leprosy control activities, together with rehabilitation of patients with nerve damage.[18] A new concern is that, while MDT is effective in treating patients, it does not always prevent them from shedding *M. leprae* in their nasal secretions and may not adequately interrupt the transmission of leprosy.[18,19] Therefore, the global community of leprosy scientists and public health experts worries that the concept of an elimination strategy requires serious rethinking.[18]

In response to these concerns, the WHO is working in collaboration with a number of partners, including Japan's Nippon Foundation and Novartis and the International Federation of Anti-Leprosy Associations (ILEP), to develop a reinforced partnership and a new sustainable strategy for leprosy control that would include incorporation of MDT into primary health care services along with physical rehabilitation.[18,19] The complexities of MDT have also led to calls for additional research and development of new and simplified control tools. This strategy includes the possible use of shortened and simplified variations of MDT to prevent the transmission of leprosy, the development of new anti-leprosy drugs based on the *M. leprae* genome completed in 2001,[20] and opportunities to integrate leprosy control with control of other diseases of poverty,[21] including the integrated package of NTD drugs (chapter 10). Early efforts to develop a leprosy vaccine are also in progress.

Summary Points: the Neglected Mycobacterial Infections

Mycobacterial Infections

- Mycobacteria are slim bacteria with unusual growth requirements and unique structural and biochemical properties that place them in their own category of microorganisms.
- TB, caused by the bacterium *M. tuberculosis*, is the best-known mycobacterial infection of humans.
- Buruli ulcer and leprosy are two highly disfiguring and stigmatizing mycobacterial NTDs occurring almost exclusively among the impoverished living in developing countries.

Buruli ulcer

- Buruli ulcer is a highly disfiguring skin infection caused by *M. ulcerans*. The name of this condition comes from a region located near the Nile River in Uganda where large numbers of cases were reported in 1962.
- Today Buruli ulcer occurs primarily in tropical regions of West Africa.
- Buruli typically strikes school-age children and manifests as a large ulcer usually appearing on the limbs.
- Although it is typically painless and rarely results in death, the ulcer of Buruli disease has a number of catastrophic consequences for the patient, including a profound socioeconomic impact and the widespread belief that witchcraft and curses play an important role in transmitting the disease.

Summary Points *(continued)*

- Buruli is either a waterborne infection or a vector-borne infection or possibly some combination of the two.
- The management and treatment of Buruli ulcer are a complex and difficult undertaking, especially in remote tropical regions.
- The most effective treatment of large ulcers requires access not only to antibiotics but also to different surgical modalities, including skin grafting.
- Because of its victims' generally remote locations and the associated disfigurement and stigma, as well as inadequate access to health care, Buruli ulcer represents a "perfect storm" of neglect.

Leprosy

- Leprosy (also known as Hansen's disease) is caused by *M. leprae*. Because of its profoundly disfiguring clinical features, there are numerous accounts of leprosy in ancient texts. Lepraphobia was extant throughout medieval Europe. In the United States, the National Hansen's Disease Center lasted for more than 100 years before closing in 1999.
- Today, as a result of widespread availability and use of MDT, the global registered prevalence of leprosy has been reduced to 224,000 cases with an estimated 259,000 new cases detected annually.
- The highest rates of the infection are presently believed to occur in Central and Southern Africa, as well as in Brazil, India, and Nepal. Most of the patients with active cases and disabled people with leprosy live in India.
- Leprosy proceeds along either one of two clinical courses. The majority of patients develop the so-called tuberculoid form. Such patients have the ability to mount strong immunological responses against *M. leprae* and, as a result, develop only localized disease. Far more severe is the lepromatous form of leprosy. These patients experience widely disseminated disease in the skin and nerves and even the eyes, nose, mouth, and bones.
- The most widely used MDT drug regimen calls for dapsone to be administered together with the antibacterial drugs rifampin and clofazimine.
- An estimated 14 million people have so far received MDT, and all but 10 of 122 countries where leprosy was once endemic have eliminated leprosy. The barriers to leprosy elimination in the remaining 10 countries are those in common with barriers preventing elimination of many other NTDs. Another problem somewhat unique to leprosy compared to other NTDs is the relative complexity of the three-drug regimen that ensures that a patient is adequately treated.

The Kinetoplastid Infections: Human African Trypanosomiasis (Sleeping Sickness), Chagas' Disease, and the Leishmaniases

> *Black shapes crouched, lay, sat between the trees, leaning against the trunk, clinging to the earth, half coming out, half effaced within the dim light, in all the attitudes of pain, abandonment, and despair … They were dying slowly … nothing but black shadows of disease and starvation, lying confusedly in the greenish gloom.*
>
> JOSEPH CONRAD, *HEART OF DARKNESS*

The kinetoplastid infections constitute a group of three major human protozoan infections caused by single-celled parasites with a flagellum and an unusual DNA-containing cell organelle known as the kinetoplastid. Like lymphatic filariasis (LF) and onchocerciasis, the kinetoplastid infections are transmitted by insect vectors. Together, the three major kinetoplastid infections of humans, human African trypanosomiasis (HAT), Chagas' disease, and leishmaniasis, kill an approximately 150,000 people annually, making them among the most lethal neglected tropical diseases (NTDs). Equally important are their poverty-promoting effects and their particular propensity to reappear in areas of conflict or postconflict turmoil, with often devastating consequences for vulnerable and migratory populations. For example, between 1988 and 1994 an estimated 100,000 perished from leishmaniasis in the western Upper Nile region of Sudan, and over the last decade in regions of war-torn Angola, the Democratic Republic of the Congo (DRC), Sudan, and Uganda, the death rate from HAT has exceeded that of HIV/AIDS.[1] Many of these deaths could have been avoided if the victims of trypanosomiasis and leishmaniasis had had access to essential medicines. However, even when the drugs are available, they are often highly toxic and can sometimes even kill patients. Most of the drugs used to treat the kinetoplastid infections are older agents which were developed in the early or middle parts of the 20th century. Because there is essentially no market in North America, Europe, or Japan for drugs to treat kinetoplastid infections, there has been little economic incentive to develop new and improved versions.

HAT

The modern history of sub-Saharan Africa is linked intimately to the transmission of HAT, also known as sleeping sickness. It is a highly lethal NTD caused by protozoan parasites in the bloodstream and central nervous system of an estimated 300,000 to 500,000 people (although some estimates are considerably higher) living in the "tsetse belt," which extends across the continent from Senegal in the west to Somalia in the east. This belt is the ecological habitat of more than 20 species of the tsetse, a biting fly of the genus *Glossina* that serves as the insect vector of HAT. Presently, the greatest numbers of HAT infections and the greatest risk of acquiring HAT occur primarily in belt areas where long-standing conflicts have thwarted public health control measures simultaneously aimed at tsetse control and human case detection and treatment.[1] In Angola, the Central African Republic (CAR), DRC, Sudan, and northern Uganda, HAT has reemerged in parallel with the past and present human-invented calamities in these countries.[1]

HAT is caused by infection with one of two subspecies of *Trypanosoma brucei*, a slender and graceful-appearing protozoan that swims in the human bloodstream with the aid of a flagellum (Color Plate 14). The graceful motion of trypanosomes as seen under a microscope results from the membrane attachment of the flagellum along the length of the parasite. The term "undulating membrane" has been used to describe this structure.

There are three major morphologically indistinguishable subspecies of *T. brucei* causing human and animal disease (Table 7.1). *T. brucei gambiense* (*T. b. gambiense*) is the cause of human sleeping sickness in West Africa (known as Gambian HAT). *T. brucei rhodesiense* (*T. b. rhodesiense*) causes HAT in East Africa (known as Rhodesian HAT).[2] A third subspecies, *T. brucei brucei* (*T. b. brucei*), does not infect humans. Instead, infection with *T. b. brucei* and other animal trypanosomes has a serious impact on the health of the rural poor in Africa because it causes a serious wasting disease in cattle known as nagana (sometimes written as n'gana), which severely reduces meat and dairy production in the region. By some estimates, 30% of sub-Saharan Africa's 150 million cattle are at risk for nagana, and the losses in milk and meat production reach an estimated US$5 billion annually.[3] Humans and cattle become infected with trypanosomes when the infective form of the parasite (known as a metacyclic trypanosome) living in the salivary glands of the female tsetse enters mammalian tissues as the fly bites (Fig. 7.1). Following inflammation at the site of

Table 7.1 The major species of HAT and animal trypanosomiasis

Disease	Parasite	Tsetse vector	Geographic distribution	Major animal reservoir of infection?
West African (Gambian) HAT	*T. b. gambiense*	*Glossina* species of the palpalis group	West Africa extending east to Sudan and parts of Uganda	No
East African (Rhodesian) HAT	*T. b. rhodesiense*	*Glossina* species of the morsitans group	East Africa (more limited distribution than *T. b. gambiense*)	Yes
Nagana (bovine trypanosomiasis)	*T. b. brucei* *T. vivax* *T. congolense*	*Glossina* species	Throughout the tsetse belt	Yes

the bite (a lesion known as a chancre), the parasites enter the lymph nodes before they eventually enter the bloodstream and multiply through asexual division as the trypomastigote form. The presence of trypanosomes in the blood is known as parasitemia. When another tsetse bites an infected person or animal with parasitemia, the trypanosomes are taken up by the fly, undergo development in the insect gut, and then migrate from the insect gut to the salivary glands. The disease is subsequently transmitted by the bite of another tsetse fly.

Scientific research conducted over the past 3 decades has shown that both humans and trypanosomes have developed some highly interesting invasion and defense mechanisms as a consequence of the evolution of the host-parasite relationship. For instance, the *T. b. brucei* subspecies causing nagana in cattle cannot survive in human blood because it is vulnerable to the toxic effects of our unique high-density liproprotein (HDL).[4] In the presence of human HDL, *T. b. brucei* trypanosomes are quickly destroyed. It is therefore possible that HDL (often referred to as "the good cholesterol") evolved in humans as a natural defense mechanism against *T. b. brucei* in addition to its role in facilitating cholesterol metabolism and in countering the effects of low-density lipoprotein (LDL) in coronary artery disease. In contrast, both *T. b. gambiense* and *T. b. rhodesiense* have evolved biochemical mechanisms to resist the trypanocidal effects of HDL. Another important survival mechanism of trypanosomes is their unique ability to evade host mammalian immune responses. Ordinarily, a human or cow would combat infectious pathogens by producing specific antibodies against them, usually within a few days or weeks after initial infection. However, trypanosomes have evolved a means of changing their surface antigens, a phenomenon known as antigenic variation, such that by the time there is a host response to the invading parasites through specific antibody production, a proportion of the trypanosomes have changed the composition of their surface antigen glycoproteins.[5] The newly masked trypanosomes are thereby rendered refractory to antibody-mediated attack. This process goes

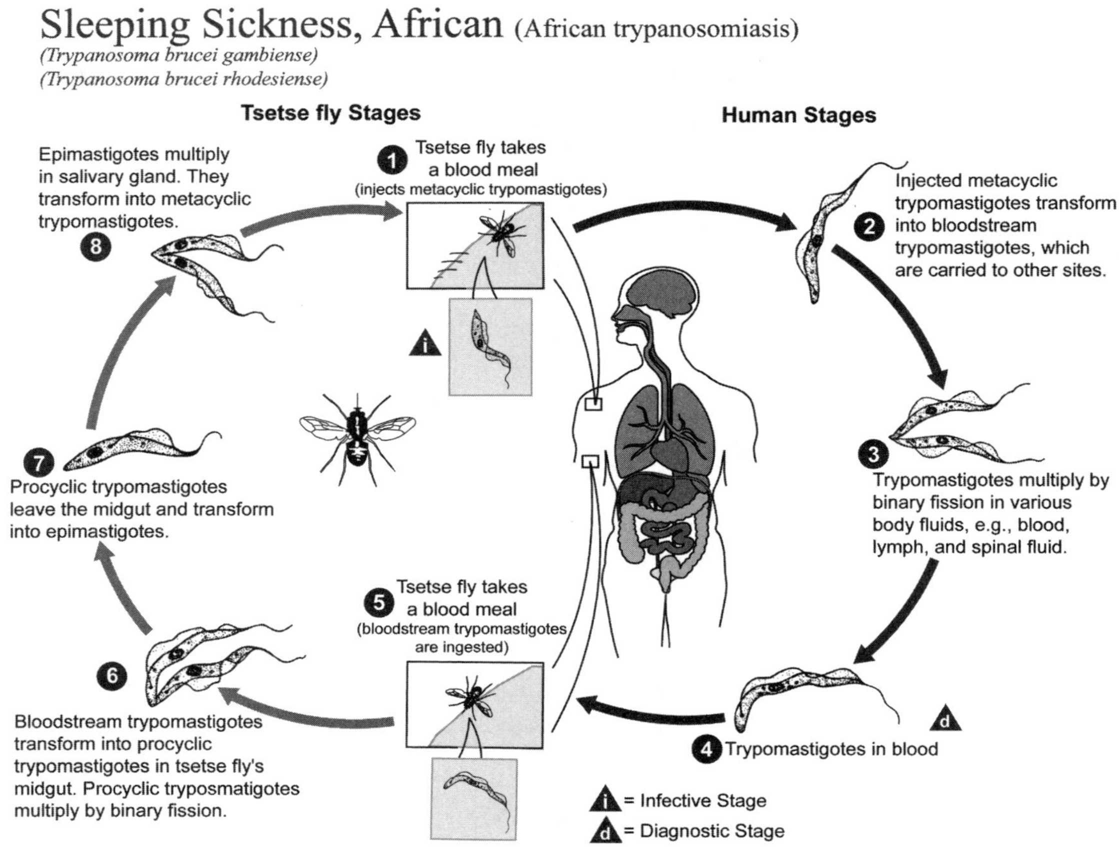

Sleeping Sickness, African (African trypanosomiasis)

(Trypanosoma brucei gambiense)
(Trypanosoma brucei rhodesiense)

Tsetse fly Stages   **Human Stages**

Epimastigotes multiply in salivary gland. They transform into metacyclic trypomastigotes.

8

1 Tsetse fly takes a blood meal (injects metacyclic trypomastigotes)

i

Injected metacyclic trypomastigotes transform into bloodstream trypomastigotes, which are carried to other sites.

2

7
Procyclic trypomastigotes leave the midgut and transform into epimastigotes.

3
Trypomastigotes multiply by binary fission in various body fluids, e.g., blood, lymph, and spinal fluid.

5 Tsetse fly takes a blood meal (bloodstream trypomastigotes are ingested)

6

Bloodstream trypomastigotes transform into procyclic trypomastigotes in tsetse fly's midgut. Procyclic tryposmatigotes multiply by binary fission.

4 Trypomastigotes in blood

d

i = Infective Stage
d = Diagnostic Stage

Figure 7.1 The life cycle of human trypanosomes and HAT (Public Health Image Library, CDC [http://phil.cdc.gov]).

on for multiple generations of parasites living in the bloodstream until they ultimately gain access to and invade the central nervous system.

There is minimal geographic overlap between the two forms of HAT—presently, Uganda is the only nation with both West and East African forms of the disease.[2] There are also pronounced differences between the clinical features of West African or Gambian HAT (*T. b. gambiense* infection) and those of East African or Rhodesian HAT (*T. b. rhodesiense* infection), as well as pronounced differences in their epidemiology and ecology. However, the ultimate outcome of the two diseases—coma and death—is the same.[2] HAT is invariably fatal unless treated.

West African HAT typically occurs around rivers, especially in areas of dense vegetation where tsetses of the *Glossina palpalis* group are abundant. The largest numbers of infections occur in war-torn regions of Angola, the CAR, southern Sudan, and the DRC. This form of HAT can last for years before the classical features of sleeping sickness appear. Early in its course, Gambian HAT presents in a fairly nonspecific way with fever, fatigue, and headache, although some telltale signs also occur, such as enlargement of the lymph nodes in the posterior region of the neck, just behind the ear, as well as swelling of the face and itching.[2] Enlargement of the lymph nodes in the neck is known as Winterbottom's sign, named after a British colonial physician who linked this finding to what he called "the Negro lethargy" while working in Sierra Leone.[6] Both anemia and endocrine disturbances also occur. This first phase of the illness lasts approximately 2 years; unless treated, this phase is inevitably followed by the sleeping sickness stage, which corresponds to invasion by the parasite of the central nervous system. In the brain and in the overlying tissues known as the meninges, the multiplying trypanosomes produce chronic inflammation (referred to as meningoencephalitis), characterized initially by severe and unrelenting headache and disturbances of gait and parkinsonism-like movements. There are also profound changes in the patient's personality, such as extreme paranoia and aggression and, between bouts of such behavior, daytime sleeping. Eventually, the patient becomes comatose and dies.

East African or Rhodesian HAT, which occurs predominantly in Kenya, Malawi, Mozambique, Tanzania, Uganda, and Zambia, has a much more rapid course, with death usually occurring within a year following the onset of early symptoms.[2] An epidemic of Rhodesian HAT in British East Africa between 1902 and 1905 may have killed as many as 250,000 people.[6] Rhodesian HAT also exhibits important differences in its epidemiology when compared with Gambian HAT. The former is transmitted by the morsitans group of *Glossina* tsetses, which preferentially feed on domestic animals (e.g., pigs, dogs, sheep, cattle, and goats) and wild game animals (such as bushbuck) rather than on humans. *Glossina morsitans* also transmits HAT primarily in woodland savanna settings rather than near rivers.[2] *T. b. rhodesiense*, unlike *T. b. gambiense*, has the ability to replicate in a wide variety of mammals, so humans are more or less accidental hosts of this parasite. In contrast, *T. b. gambiense* is probably a parasite exclusively of humans. We will see below how the fact that Rhodesian HAT is primarily a zoonosis, i.e., a disease transmitted from animals to humans, has important implications for controlling epidemics of this disease.

Because of its dramatic clinical features, inevitable lethality, and ability to decimate entire African villages, sleeping sickness has made an indelible imprint on the history of sub-Saharan Africa. In terms of its impact on colonial history, sleeping sickness did much to thwart European ambitions on the African continent, and the colonial administrations of the United Kingdom, as well as of Belgium, France, Germany, and Portugal, responded to this threat by investing a considerable component of their medical activities in its study. At least as much as any other single disease, it was HAT that stimulated colonial European governments to commission a first generation of schools of tropical medicine in Antwerp (Belgium), Basel (Switzerland), Hamburg (Germany), Lisbon (Portugal), and Liverpool and London (England) during the last decade of the 19th century and in the first decades of the 20th century. The founding of these schools mostly in European seaports reflected the impact of HAT and other tropical diseases on returning seamen and practitioners of other occupations connected with vital shipping interests.[7] Sir Alfred Lewis Jones, the founder of the Liverpool School of Tropical Medicine, was one of Liverpool's leading businessmen who invested heavily in the shipping trade with West Africa.[7]

It was during this period that the toll of sleeping sickness in sub-Saharan Africa began to be widely appreciated, particularly with colonial expansion into the Belgian Congo, the same location where Joseph Conrad in *Heart of Darkness* placed his abandoned individuals presumably suffering from sleeping sickness.[7] Working in Zululand (the site of present-day KwaZulu-Natal Province of South Africa) in 1894, Surgeon-Captain David Bruce, a Scottish bacteriologist working in the British Army, first identified trypanosomes from cattle with nagana and demonstrated that he could reproduce a wasting disease in dogs by injecting them with the same microorganisms; a year later he identified the tsetse as the natural vector for nagana.[6] In 1902, John Everett Dutton of the Liverpool School of Tropical Medicine provided one of the first descriptions of a human trypanosome from a seaman who worked on steamships on the Gambia River.[6] A reproduction of Dutton's original watercolor drawing of what he named *T. gambiense* is shown in Color Plate 15. Three years after his discovery, Dutton died from relapsing fever (an unrelated bacterial infection) while working in the Belgian Congo. Today, there stands a church in Dutton's home village of Bunbury, Cheshire (outside Liverpool), with a stained-glass panel commemorating both Dutton and the accomplishments of the Liverpool School.[6,7] Subsequently, while investigating a sleeping sickness outbreak in Uganda as part of a sleeping sickness commission sponsored by the Royal Society of London, David Bruce, together with Aldo Castellani, demonstrated that this human trypanosome was also transmitted by tsetses.[6] Bruce also determined that the organism causing Rhodesian HAT was transmitted from animals to humans.[6]

Concurrent with the activities of the British at the turn of the 20th century, there were also efforts in France, Germany, Switzerland, and England to develop new treatments for HAT. As early as 1858, the explorer David Livingstone was using arsenic to treat tsetse bites, and in 1902 Alphonse Laveran, the French codiscoverer of the malaria parasite, found that sodium arsenite was a potential treatment for HAT.[8] Shortly thereafter, it was discovered that if arsenic was modified by chemically linking it with an organic compound, its toxicity diminished considerably.[8] In 1907, Paul Ehrlich, the father of chemotherapy, synthesized and accurately characterized atoxyl, one of the first such organified arsenic compounds.[8] Ehrlich was a Prussian Jew who worked initially with Robert Koch in Berlin and then moved to Frankfurt, where he headed the Royal Institute for Experimental Therapy.[8] Subsequently, at the Liverpool School, Anton Breinl showed that atoxyl could be developed as a treatment for trypanosomiasis in laboratory animals,[7] and although the compound was extremely toxic, this discovery led to the development of a related arsenic-containing compound, melarsoprol.[8] A second organified arsenic compound, tryparsamide, was also developed around this period at the Rockefeller Institute for Medical Research, the forerunner of today's Rockefeller University.[8] These discoveries laid the foundation for the development and testing of melarsoprol, which became the first successful arsenical drug for sleeping sickness. First developed by Ernst Friedheim (1899–1989), a Swiss physician and chemist, melarsoprol has a better safety profile than does the first generation of arsenicals, atoxyl and tryparsamide.[8] However, because of its arsenic component, melarsoprol is still considered highly toxic, and even today up to 10% of patients undergoing treatment for sleeping sickness with the drug either die or experience a severe toxic reaction known as posttreatment reactive encephalopathy (PTRE).[9] Sadly, despite its toxicity, melarsoprol still remains one of only a few drugs available for the treatment of central nervous system HAT.

In addition to melarsoprol, there are two other drugs, pentamidine and suramin (neither of which is an arsenical), still in widespread use for the earlier stage of HAT (prior to parasite invasion of the central nervous system). Both drugs were developed even before melarsoprol. Discovered in 1916, suramin is a derivative of the dye trypan red; by noting that many dyes bound selectively to microorganisms, Paul Ehrlich had earlier pioneered the concept that they could also be developed into chemotherapeutic agents.[8] Subsequently, the drug pentamidine was discovered in 1936.[8] Therefore, almost our entire pharmacopoeia for HAT relies on drugs that are more than 50 years old!

Since 2005, the entire genome of *T. brucei* has been sequenced, and it is theoretically possible to mine this information in order to develop a new generation of antitrypanosomal drugs.[10] You might ask how it can be that we use such old-fashioned drugs with relatively high levels of toxicity, when it is possible to develop safer and more effective drugs. There are a number of reasons for this overall absence in research and development activities, but primarily it is because HAT is an NTD and there is no commercial incentive for drug companies to develop and test new compounds. We saw previously in the chapters about onchocerciasis, LF, and trachoma that the large pharmaceutical companies are prepared to donate drugs, but it is another matter altogether for any publicly held company to convince its shareholders to launch and invest in a discovery program for guaranteed money-losing products. The problem of access to essential medicines for HAT is therefore twofold: first, the existing drugs are highly toxic and often not available, and second, there is no incentive to develop new drugs. Another example of this second problem is illustrated by a newer agent for HAT known as eflornithine. Eflornithine was originally developed and tested as a new anticancer drug, but it was subsequently abandoned for that purpose. Although it might have failed as a breakthrough against cancer, during the 1990s it was discovered that eflornithine was effective against the central nervous system stage of Gambian HAT. This discovery was considered a breakthrough because eflornithine was the first drug for late-stage sleeping sickness that did not contain toxic arsenic. However, without a commercially viable market, there were no incentives for pharmaceutical companies to develop eflornithine for use in sub-Saharan Africa. In 2001, the French nonprofit organization Médecins Sans Frontièrs (MSF) (Doctors Without Borders) together with the World Health Organization successfully lobbied to encourage the pharmaceutical company Sanofi Aventis to manufacture eflornithine and make it widely available in Africa. In a landmark agreement, Sanofi-Pasteur also agreed to produce pentamidine and melarsoprol. Later (in chapter 11), we will also see how new product development partnerships—such as the Geneva-based Drugs for

Neglected Diseases Initiative (DNDi), a partnership of several organizations including MSF; the Oswaldo Cruz Foundation in Brazil; the Indian Council for Medical Research; the Kenya Medical Research Institute; the Ministry of Health of Malaysia; the Institut Pasteur in France; and the Special Programme on Tropical Disease Research (TDR)—are developing and clinically testing additional antitrypanosomal drugs. Both DNDi (http://www.dndi.org) and smaller academically based research institutions, such as the Sandler Center for Basic Research in Parasitic Diseases at the University of California, San Francisco, and the Seattle Biomedical Research Institute, are using highly innovative, high-throughput approaches based on the genome of *T. brucei* to discover new antitrypanosomal drugs, while a Gates Foundation-sponsored consortium based at the University of North Carolina is reconfiguring a drug developed to treat fungal infections in order to target HAT.[11] Also in place are efforts to reduce the toxicity of existing drugs, including melarsoprol, by reducing the amount that needs to be administered through supplementation with the compound nifurtimox.[12] Therefore, there is a high level of excitement that several new drugs for HAT could be developed in the coming decade.

By the middle of the 20th century, tremendous progress in the control and prevention of HAT had been made in both West and East Africa. However, based on the different epidemiological patterns of the two forms of HAT, a different approach was required to control each form of the disease.[13] Because Gambian HAT is exclusively a human disease (i.e., no significant animal reservoir is involved in disease transmission), the major approach for control has been to conduct massive screenings for *T. b. gambiense* infection and then treat infected patients. Throughout the first part of the 20th century in French and Belgian colonial West Africa, tens of millions of people were screened by mobile field teams. If they were found to be positive, they were treated with tryparsamide. Through this activity, the human reservoir of trypanosomes was depleted and transmission was interrupted. The French physician and scientist Eugene Jamot (1879–1937) is largely credited with developing this strategy.[13,14] While working in Cameroon, for instance, Jamot is believed to have reduced the incidence of Gambian HAT by 300-fold. For this work, Jamot was nominated for the Nobel Prize.[13,14] In contrast, because East African HAT has a significant animal reservoir for transmission and *T. b. rhodesiense* trypanosomes can be found in abundance in cattle and bushbuck, the Jamot method would not be expected to work. One draconian practice during the early 20th century in British-held East Africa was forced human resettlement away from regions inhabited by bushbuck and other animals.[6] Today, in eastern Uganda, the husband-wife team of Ian Maudlin and Sue Welburn has determined that 18% of domestic cattle harbor *T. b. rhodesiense* and represent a significant reservoir of human-infective trypanosomes. By treating infected cattle either with antitrypanosomal drugs or pour-on insecticides, they are exploring the possibility that this approach could interrupt the human transmission of HAT. Both West and East African approaches benefit from vector control methods, including the use of baited tsetse traps and widespread application of insecticides.[13]

Compared to mass drug administrations for NTDs such as the soil-transmitted helminth infections, schistosomiasis, LF, onchocerciasis, and trachoma, the control practices for both Gambian HAT and Rhodesian HAT are extremely labor-intensive. Therefore, while it is often feasible to control Gambian HAT through case identification and treatment or Rhodesian HAT by targeting animal reservoirs, when conditions make it difficult to apply these methods, it does not take much to derail public health control measures for HAT and allow a recrudescence of the disease. This is exactly what has happened in many conflict and postconflict states of sub-Saharan Africa. One of the better-documented examples of a truly horrific humanitarian catastrophe is represented by the nation of Angola.[15] With a total area of almost 500,000 sq. mi. (and 12 million people), Angola is one of the largest countries in Africa. During the years between 1926 and 1952, a series of aggressive campaigns were launched to control Gambian HAT. Based on the classic Jamot model of case identification and treatment, an important component of the Angolan control program was the Brigade for Pentamidinization, in which infected individuals were identified and were treated with the antitrypanosomal drug pentamidine.[14] In the year prior to Angola's independence in 1975, only three cases in the country could be found. Unfortunately, this was the beginning of the end. Starting in 1976, clashes between UNITA (National Union for the Total Independence of Angola) and the Soviet-backed Marxist state of the MPLA (Movement for the Liberation of Angola) ignited almost 30 years of war.[15] A major hurdle to implementing screening measures was inaccessibility as a result of insecurity and land mines. HAT-infected patients were unable to reach diagnosis and treatment centers, while at the same time, mobile health units could not travel.[15] In addition, there was massive looting of technical equipment, including drugs and microscopes. As a result, the number of people screened for HAT went from a high of 12 million (the entire population) during the 1950s to about only 150,000 by 1998.[15] By this time almost 7,000 cases had been detected, but presumably there were at least 10 times that, according to studies in Uganda indicating that an estimated 12 deaths caused by sleeping sickness go undetected for every one reported.[16]

During the war years, only the Catholic Church was permitted to conduct cross-border initiatives through ANGOTRIP, an organization created for HAT control in the region.[15] At local health centers established in regions of HAT endemicity in the northwestern part of the country, a diagnosis was established by palpating neck lymph nodes (Winterbottom's sign) or by identifying trypanosomes in the blood by microscopy, as well as by using a serological method that detects antitrypanosomal antibodies. Treatments of infected patients were conducted either with pentamidine or melarsoprol, depending on whether there was central nervous system involvement. Between 1996 and 2001, ANGOTRIP screened almost 200,000 patients and achieved a substantial reduction in HAT mortality.[15] It has been suggested that the death of UNITA leader Jonas Savimbi in 2002 may help to restore some semblance of public health infrastructure.[15] Sadly, there are similar stories of Gambian HAT's resurgence because of warfare in the DRC, Sudan, and elsewhere, while in East

Africa, there remains a similar vulnerability to epidemic outbreaks of Rhodesian HAT. For instance, around the Lake Victoria basin, epidemics killing tens of thousands of people have occurred periodically, including a major outbreak in Uganda during the 1980s.[16,17] The relationship between "conflict and contagion" remains a major theme of HAT's reemergence in sub-Saharan Africa.[18]

Chagas' disease (American trypanosomiasis)

American trypanosomiasis is also named Chagas' disease in honor of Carlos Chagas, who as a young Brazilian physician in 1909 identified *Trypanosoma cruzi* (named after his mentor, Oswaldo Cruz) as the causative agent and then went on to elucidate the entire life cycle of the infection.[19] Except for being caused by a trypanosome, American trypanosomiasis bears very little resemblance to HAT in either its clinical features or its epidemiology. An estimated 8 to 9 million suffer from Chagas' disease,[20] an insect vector-borne infection occurring almost exclusively among the very poorest inhabitants of Latin America. The major foci of endemic Chagas' disease occur in Central America; the Andean region comprising Colombia, Ecuador, Peru, and Venezuela (DNA from *T. cruzi* has been detected in the mummified remains of people from this region, especially Peru and northern Chile, from as far back as 2000 BCE);[6] and in a region of South America known as the Southern Cone, which includes Argentina, Bolivia, Brazil, Chile, Paraguay, and Uruguay.[20] Throughout these regions of endemicity in the Americas, Chagas' disease continues to be a significant cause of chronic heart disease. In addition, cases of Chagas' disease now occur in the Amazon region and Mexico, and there is even concern that it has emerged in the United States, possibly through contamination of our blood supply with *T. cruzi*. Through an innovative vector control program known as the Southern Cone Initiative or INCOSUR (Iniciativa de Salud del Cono Sur), there have been dramatic gains in reducing the prevalence of Chagas' disease in this region.[21] Therefore, there is some optimism that through vector control Chagas' disease could be eliminated in the Southern Cone and elsewhere in the coming decades. However, just as there are important differences between the East and West African forms of HAT, there are also some regional differences in the geographic variants of Chagas' disease. Of particular importance is an endemic focus in Central America, where, because of the unique ecology of the infection and its vector, there are significant concerns that Chagas' disease may be difficult to eliminate.

Imagine a large cockroach-like bug endowed with the ability to suck blood. The vector transmitting *T. cruzi* trypanosomes is the triatomine bug, known locally as the assassin bug, kissing bug, *vinchuca* (*benchuca*), or *barbeiro* (Fig. 7.2). Triatomine bugs operate as rural cousins of the cockroach, typically living in the crevices of walls and thatch of low-quality dwellings in the rural areas of the Americas. At night they leave the safety of their crevices and thatch, often dropping down on their sleeping victims in order to feed on blood. In his travel journals from Argentina, Charles Darwin—who in his later years suffered from a variety of ailments which some authors have attributed to the

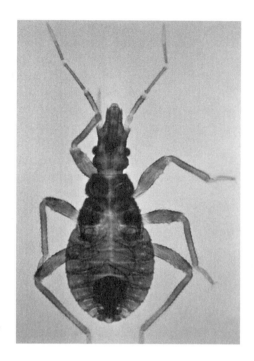

Figure 7.2 Triatomine bug (Public Health Image Library, CDC [http://phil.cdc.gov]).

chronic consequences of Chagas' disease—provided an excellent description of a vinchuca and its voracious appetite for blood:[22]

> At night I experienced an attack (for it deserves no less a name) of benchuca … the great black bug of the pampas. It is most disgusting to feel soft wing-less insects, about an inch long, crawling over one's body. Before sucking they are quite thin but afterwards they become round and bloated with blood, and in this state are easily crushed. One which I caught … was very empty. When placed on a table, and though surrounded by people, if a finger was presented, the bold insect would immediately protrude its sucker, make a charge, and if allowed, draw blood. No pain was caused by the wound. It was curious to watch its body during the act of sucking, as in less than ten minutes it changed from being as flat as a wafer to a globular form.

The possibility that the triatomine bug could transmit American trypanosomiasis was demonstrated by Carlos Chagas. As a young physician and a member of one of Brazil's first biomedical research institutes, the Institute of Experimental Pathology of Manguinhos (later named Instituto Oswaldo Cruz and now a major component of FIOCRUZ [the Oswaldo Cruz Foundation], Brazil's largest and most extensive biomedical and research organization devoted to infectious diseases and other conditions), Chagas had developed a reputation for his ability to organize and lead antimalaria campaigns in the interior of the country.[19] While he was on assignment, a railway company engineer brought to the young Chagas's attention the vinchucas inhabiting the poor dwellings of the region and their nocturnal biting behavior. Chagas began to examine vinchucas and identified trypanosomes, which he named in honor of Oswaldo Cruz, his institute director.[19] He subsequently found a trypanosome in the blood of a 22-month-old girl named Bernice who was suffering from fever with enlargement of the liver, spleen, and lymph nodes, as well as facial edema (swelling of the face). He also identified the trypanosomes in a cat that lived in the same house. Ultimately, Bernice recovered from her acute illness, and 52 years later (27 years after the death of Chagas), Bernice was rediscovered as a grandmother of three living on a farm in Minas Gerais State. Blood tests conducted at the major university teaching hospital at that time subsequently confirmed a diagnosis of Chagas' disease. Bernice ultimately died in 1981 at the age of 73.[19]

Humans become infected with *T. cruzi* in an interesting way (Fig. 7.3). Unlike metacyclic African trypanosomes, which live in the insect salivary glands and enter through a bite, the metacyclic American trypanosome lives in the hindgut of the triatomine bug. While working in Brazil around the same time as Chagas, the eminent French parasitologist Emile Brumpt

Figure 7.3 Life cycle of *T. cruzi* and Chagas' disease (Public Health Image Library, CDC [http://phil.cdc.gov]).

Trypanosomiasis, American (Chagas disease)
(Trypanosoma cruzi)

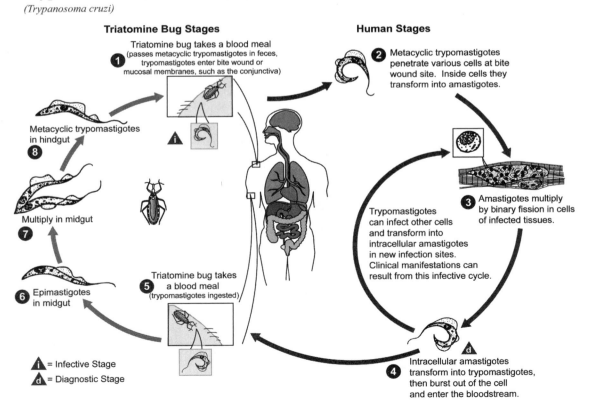

demonstrated that *T. cruzi* infection first occurs by the process of autoinoculation. This transmission phenomenon occurs when the triatomine bug defecates as it feeds; during sleep, the unsuspecting victim of the assassin bug rubs the trypanosome-infected bug feces into either the puncture wound caused by the bug or the mucous membranes of the eyes or mouth. Once the metacyclic trypanosomes invade the mucous membranes, they continue to behave quite differently from *T. brucei*. Rather than invade the bloodstream immediately and multiply as the trypomastigote form, the metacyclic *T. cruzi* trypomastigotes exhibit the ability to invade cells and multiply as intracellular pathogens.[23] Initially, this stage of invasion results in inflammation near the site of entry, causing swelling around the eye and face (known as Romana's sign) or some other region of the skin, where it is known as a chagoma. Once inside cells, the parasite replicates as a rounded, so-called amastigote form, but subsequently the cells burst and release a new round of trypomastigote forms of the parasite, which then invade the bloodstream before besieging multiple organs. Initially, organ invasion results in acute Chagas' disease associated with fever, headache, enlargement of the spleen and liver, and facial or generalized edema.[24] During this stage of the illness, it is sometimes possible to identify trypanosomes in the blood. Acute Chagas' disease can also cause inflammation of the heart (myocarditis), which has a high fatality rate because it can cause conduction disturbances in the heart or even heart failure.

Following this acute phase of the illness, many patients recover and remain asymptomatic over a period of years before entering a new phase of *T. cruzi* infection known as the chronic phase. This syndrome occurs in roughly 30% of patients who previously experienced acute Chagas' disease.[24] In the chronically affected patients, there is a severe disturbance of the electrical system of the heart leading to arrhythmias, palpitations, chest pain, difficulties with breathing on exertion, and fainting.[24] In some of these patients, there are a profound enlargement of the heart and distortion of its architecture, a condition known as cardiomyopathy. Over time, cardiomyopathy can lead to heart failure, aneurysms of the heart wall, and even sudden death. In addition to the heart changes, some patients also develop a curious disorder of their colon and esophagus in which both organs lose their tone and become grossly enlarged. Megacolon and megaesophagus are associated with regurgitation, pain on swallowing, and severe constipation. Discovery of the link between megacolon and megaesophagus (and even cardiomyopathy) and Chagas' disease has been attributed to the work of Fritz Koberle in the 1960s.[6,25] A number of hypotheses have been advanced to explain the mechanisms by which long-standing *T. cruzi* infections lead to cardiomyopathy and megacolon and megaesophagus.[25] These hypotheses are controversial because it is not clear whether these maladies result from the continuous low-grade presence of *T. cruzi* parasites in the heart and other organs or whether host immune responses are responsible. An important component of the chronic phase is thought to be an abnormality of the autonomic nervous system that controls both the heart and the gastrointestinal tract, again from either parasite invasion or autoimmunity.

The treatment of the chronic complications of Chagas' disease requires complex modalities. Chagas' cardiomyopathy is treated with antiarrhythmia drugs and pacemakers. However, for severe disease, sometimes only heart transplantation is effective. Not surprisingly, a generation of Latin American cardiac surgeons has become adept at this procedure. Surgery is also frequently required for the gastrointestinal complications. For acute Chagas' disease, there are two antitrypanosomal drugs when they are available, including nifurtimox (also used for the treatment of HAT) and benznidazole (not to be confused with the benzimidazole anthelmintics [mebendazole and albendazole] used for soil-transmitted helminth infections). Unfortunately, many patients with acute Chagas' disease are not identified in time for effective treatment, while the few who are diagnosed appropriately require 1 to 2 months of daily doses of these drugs. There is even considerable controversy about whether these drugs have a significant impact on the disease. For example, in most patients the organisms persist despite treatment, and for many, treatment does not prevent severe heart lesions or other long-term complications. These sad facts, coupled with the high acute and chronic toxicities of nifurtimox and benznidazole, suggest an urgent need for new anti-*T. cruzi* drugs.[24] The recent completion of the *T. cruzi* genome[26] should in theory lead to the development of new drugs, but the limited commercial markets have restricted these activities to just a handful of product development partnerships such as DNDi and others as outlined above for HAT.

There are no simple preventive chemotherapy approaches for the control of Chagas' disease, nor is it practical to apply wide-scale case detection and management with antitrypanosomal drugs such as what occurred with the pentamidization campaigns against HAT launched in the 20th century. Nevertheless, the INCOSUR initiative has had great success in controlling Chagas' disease in the Southern Cone through widespread insect control.[21] In this region of South America, *Triatoma infestans* is the major assassin bug vector of Chagas' disease. Because this species of assassin bug lives exclusively inside the poor dwellings of the region, it is possible to reduce infestation by residual spraying with pyrethroid insecticides.[21] This strategy also includes applications of insecticides in chicken houses and other dwellings located near the home, combined with additional spraying of any reinfested houses.[21] In areas of the Southern Cone where *T. infestans* is responsible for transmission of Chagas' disease, there has been a dramatic decrease in transmission in Argentina, Brazil, Chile, Paraguay, and Uruguay. Elimination of the disease has now been certified in Chile and Uruguay, as well as in four provinces of Argentina, 10 states in Brazil, and one state in Paraguay.[21] Since Bolivia is the poorest member state of the Southern Cone, its elimination efforts are still in an earlier stage. INCOSUR therefore represents one of the very best examples of cooperative programs between Latin American nations.

In Central America and elsewhere, the elimination of Chagas' disease through large-scale residual spraying has not been as straightforward. Efforts to reproduce INCOSUR's successes through a Central American initiative known as IPCA (Iniciativa de los paises de Centroamerica) have been complicated by the fact that *Triatoma dimidiata* and *Rhodnius prolixus*, rather than *T. infestans*, are the major vectors of Chagas' disease in this region. Unlike *T. infestans*, *T. dimidiata* can live in the palm trees surrounding the houses, and there are no effective methods for insecticide spraying of palms.[21] Therefore, control efforts require multiple sprayings each time the vectors enter households. This problem makes community-based surveillance, including case detection and management, all the more important.[21,27]

With the exception of Venezuela, efforts in the Andean region have not progressed nearly as far as in the Southern Cone, with baseline surveys only beginning in many regions. As a long-term measure, it is theoretically possible to develop a Chagas' disease vaccine, but the development testing of a new generation of antipoverty vaccines remains elusive because of the challenges of taking on product development for the world's poorest people.

When I travel to Central America, it is always amazing for me to realize that from Miami or Houston I can reach within just a few hours many regions of Central America where one of the most important neglected diseases of poverty remains endemic. On most days, I can reach the Chagas-endemic regions of Honduras faster than I can reach the West Coast of the United States. On several occasions I have awakened either in New Haven or Washington, DC in the morning, and by late in the afternoon I am making pediatric rounds in the children's wards of the public hospitals in Central America, where I can see sick children with Chagas' disease and other NTDs as well as malnutrition. While so much attention is now being paid to sub-Saharan Africa, it is a sad state of affairs that some of our closest neighboring countries cannot benefit from the very best that Western biotechnology has to offer.

Leishmaniasis

Leishmaniasis is a serious parasitic disease affecting an estimated 12 million poor people in developing countries. There are two major forms of the disease—visceral leishmaniasis (VL; also known as kala-azar) is a disseminated infection affecting multiple organs, including the liver, spleen, blood, and bone marrow, and cutaneous leishmaniasis (CL) is an ulcerative and often highly disfiguring chronic skin infection. A less common third, mucocutaneous form (MCL) is also found in Central and South America. Ancient accounts of leishmaniasis were recorded by the Persian physician and philosopher Avicenna (Abū Alī al-Ḥusayn ibn Abd Allāh ibn Sīnā) in the 10th century, and there are several descriptions of the illness going as far back as the 7th century BCE.[6] Annually, leishmaniasis strikes approximately 1.5 to 2 million people (and causes 70,000 deaths) in a wide geographic range across the tropics and subtropics.[3] For all forms of the disease, access to essential medicines and the toxicity of the existing antileishmania drugs remain major obstacles to public health control. According to disease burden estimates based on healthy life years lost from premature death or disability (disability-adjusted life years, or DALYs), leishmaniasis is the most important protozoan infection of humans after malaria. Leishmaniasis has also been noted as an important opportunistic infection in patients with underlying HIV/AIDS.

Except for a small focus of the disease in southern Europe, leishmaniasis occurs almost exclusively in low- and middle-income countries. Most of the cases of CL occur in Central Asia and the Middle East (especially Afghanistan, Algeria, Iran, Pakistan, Saudi Arabia, and Syria) or in the Americas (especially Brazil and Peru), while the highest rates of VL occur on the Indian subcontinent (India, Bangladesh, and Nepal) and in Sudan and Brazil.[28,29] In these regions, poor rural housing conditions such as cracked walls and earthen floors allow the sandfly vectors that transmit both VL and CL to flourish, while in some urban areas with poor sanitation, the uncollected garbage provides additional sandfly niches, because it promotes habitats for stray dogs, which can sometimes serve as animal reservoirs of the infection.[30] Another important link between leishmaniasis and poverty is the limited access for the poorest people in Asia, Africa, and India to essential medicines. Today, our lack of effective medicines and access to populations affected by leishmaniasis are the greatest obstacles to control. This problem is particularly true for women, who are severely stigmatized as a result of this disfiguring infection and as a result are often denied access to both health care and treatments. Limited access may account for the striking finding that the disease burden of leishmaniasis as measured in DALYs is higher for women than for men.[30]

Another important risk factor for leishmaniasis is conflict. Just as interruption of public health measures such as case identification and treatment and vector control led to a resurgence of HAT in Angola, the DRC, Sudan, and elsewhere, in 1988, 5 years into a renewed conflict in southern Sudan, a massive epidemic of VL occurred in the western Upper Nile Province of Sudan, particularly among war refugees who settled along the Sudanese-Ethiopian border.[31] The major reasons for the epidemic of VL were interruption of residual spraying for malaria (which is also effective at controlling sandfly populations), movement of military personnel from areas of Ethiopia where VL was also endemic, and malnutrition among the refugees, which may have increased their susceptibility to infection.[31] Up to 30,000 people died from VL in 1988, and another 19,000 patients were treated in emergency centers set up by Médecins Sans Frontières between 1989 and 1995.[31] Some estimates suggest that between 1984 and 1994, approximately 100,000 deaths occurred among an estimated 280,000 infected people.[31] Thus, the conflict in Sudan has allowed at least three serious NTDs to flourish—HAT, trachoma, and VL—on top of the soil-transmitted helminthiases and schistosomiasis endemic to the region.

Both VL and CL are also common diseases in patients with HIV/AIDS. There is a unique HIV-associated focus of VL in southern Europe (where approximately 2,000 cases of coinfection have been reported) and elsewhere, especially in Brazil.

There are multiple species of *Leishmania* parasites that cause either VL or CL (Table 7.2). Leishmaniasis is transmitted by the bite of small and delicate-appearing sandflies, which inoculate flagellated forms of the parasite (known as promastigotes) into the skin (Fig. 7.4).[29,32] What then happens is remarkable.

Table 7.2 Simplified summary of the human leishmaniases[a]

Disease	Major Old World species	Major Old World geographic distribution	Major New World species	Major New World geographic distribution
VL	*L. donovani*	Sudan and Indian subcontinent (Nepal and Bangladesh)	*L. chagasi*	Brazil
	L. infantum	Southern Europe		
CL	*L. tropica* and *L. major*	Afghanistan, Algeria, Iran, Pakistan, Saudi Arabia, Sudan, Syria	Numerous species	Peru, Brazil, Central America
MCL			*L. braziliensis*	Bolivia, Brazil, Peru, Central America

[a]Based on information from Alvar et al., 2006a.

Rather than avoid being ingested and killed by macrophages—professional killer cells designed by our bodies to ward off infectious agents—the *Leishmania* parasites actually attract these cells so that they can be ingested by them more efficiently. Once inside macrophages, the parasites multiply as amastigote forms, which actually thrive and multiply in a toxic environment of microbicidal enzymes and chemicals that would ordinarily kill almost any other microorganism. Eventually, the macrophages rupture, releasing new amastigotes which in turn invade new macrophages. In the case of CL, the infected macrophages and amastigotes remain in the skin, while in VL, the macrophages travel to the liver, spleen, and bone marrow, where these infected cells release new rounds of amastigotes and cause significant systemic effects.[29] In humans, therefore, the kinetoplastid trypanosomes causing HAT live an entirely extracellular existence, while American trypanosomes live both intracellularly and extracellularly and *Leishmania* parasites are almost entirely intracellular.

In the early stages, the clinical features of CL resemble those of Buruli ulcer, beginning as a nodule and then over a period of weeks to months degenerating into an ulcer. The ulcer, which is known by a number of different names depending on its geographic location (such as Baghdad boil, Delhi boil, Aleppo evil, Balkh Sore, and oriental sore) has a cratered center and raised margins (Fig. 7.5). The term "pizza-like" is frequently used. With time, most CL lesions self-heal, but often not before they produce a disfiguring scar. MCL is a major variant of CL in which ulceration erodes the cartilage of the nose to produce horrific destruction of the face.

In places such as Afghanistan or India, a CL lesion or scar can have catastrophic social consequences. The stigma of CL, like the stigma of many NTDs, is particularly severe for girls and women of reproductive age. For instance, in Afghanistan, even though CL is not transmitted by contact between people (it requires the sandfly vector), mothers with CL are prevented from touching their children and young women with CL are unable to marry. In Colombia, husbands abandon their infected wives, and in Bangladesh, the husband's family will not pay for medical care.[30]

Leishmaniasis
(Leishmania spp.)

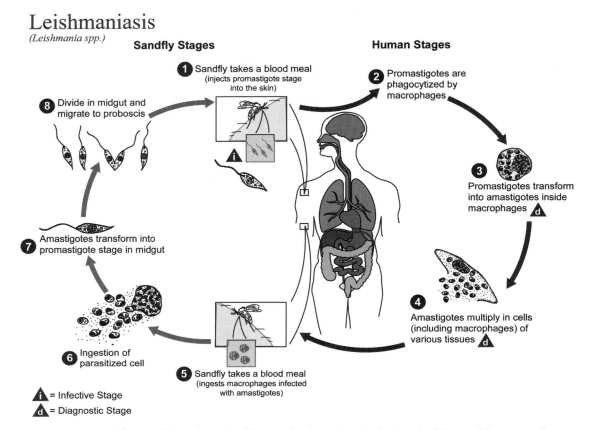

Figure 7.4 Life cycle of human leishmaniasis infection (Public Health Image Library, CDC [http://phil.cdc.gov]).

Because it affects multiple internal organs and the blood, VL produces a far more extensive illness, manifesting as high fever, with fever spikes several times a day, night sweats, loss of appetite, and severe weight loss proceeding over a period of months.[29] In many regions VL has a predilection for young children, who often have a surprising level of energy and activity despite their severe and profound level of disease. The large number of parasites in the bone marrow of these children results in an inability of the patient to produce both white blood cells and red blood cells. As a result, infected children and adults experience pancytopenia, a decrease in their circulating blood cell counts leading to anemia and other blood abnormalities. Their livers and spleens become dramatically enlarged. When cases of VL are exported to the United States, such children are often erroneously diagnosed as having advanced leukemias or lymphomas. In some patients their skin becomes dark; in India and elsewhere, VL is sometimes named kala-azar, meaning black fever.[29] Among patients who died from VL in the Sudanese epidemic during the late 1980s, and early 1990s, the most important risk factors for death were age (the very young and the

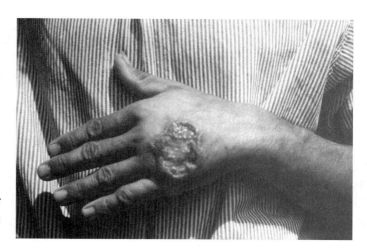

Figure 7.5 The "pizza-like" lesion of CL (Public Health Image Library, CDC [http://phil.cdc.gov]).

very old), duration of illness greater than 5 months, severe anemia and malnutrition, a large spleen, and a high parasite load in the tissues.[31] Working in India in 1899, the eminent malariologist Sir Ronald Ross thought that VL was a severe form of malaria. It was not until a few years later that William Leishman, a Scottish army doctor, and Charles Donovan, a medical school professor at Madras University, found the cause of kala-azar.[6]

Both CL and VL are treatable infections, but many of the drugs used produce severe toxicities, and in many cases they are not available. For the treatment of central nervous system HAT, we learned about continuing reliance on highly toxic arsenical compounds even though it is possible to design a new generation of antitrypanosomal drugs. The situation for leishmaniasis is not much better—rather than poisoning our patients with arsenic, we instead poison them with the heavy metal antimony! In most of the world, compounds containing antimony are still the treatment of choice for leishmaniasis. Usually, a month of daily injections with the antimony-containing compound stibogluconate is required for the treatment of VL. Such treatments are expensive both in terms of actual money and the precious time that patients lose from work. Estimates for a course of treatment range from US$30 to US$1,500 just for the medicines, and when the overall costs of lost productivity and impact on affected families are measured, the results are staggering. For instance, in Nepal, the median cost for one VL patient is equivalent to the yearly median per capita income.[30] The treatment of CL also requires multiple toxic injections, and in that regard it is questionable whether there is sufficient therapeutic benefit in administering the drug rather than allowing the cutaneous ulcers to self-heal. Better clinical trials that accurately measure cure rates (in terms of both clinical response rates and reduction of parasite loads) are required for both forms of leishmaniasis.

There are alternative approaches to treat CL and VL, which include the use of a medicine known as amphotericin B that was developed primarily for the treatment of opportunistic fungal infections in immunocompromised patients with cancer and other serious disorders. Although in many cases a single dose of a new lipid formulation of amphotericin B is often effective for the treatment of VL, the hundreds of dollars for even a single dose render the drug prohibitively expensive in Bihar State in India (where there is widespread stibogluconate resistance) and other low-income areas. Similarly, there is a new oral drug for VL known as miltefosine, which would be ideal for treating poor people with VL in an outpatient setting, but it too is often too expensive. Therefore, the poorest patients with VL must endure lengthy and toxic treatments with antimony-containing medicines or, in many cases, have no access at all to essential medicine. At least two major nonprofit organizations, the DNDi and the Institute for One World Health, are working to develop and test new and less toxic drugs, which can be given in brief therapeutic courses suitable for resource-poor settings. Through such efforts, the drug paromomycin was approved by the Drug Controller-General of India. A single treatment course with this drug is estimated to be less than US$10 per patient.[33]

Efforts to control leishmaniasis worldwide are complicated by the complex epidemiology of both VL and CL.[28] In some areas of the world, such as in Brazil and southern Europe, sandflies can transmit leishmaniasis from dogs to humans. The control of so-called zoonotic leishmaniasis is typically accomplished by targeting these animals through culling or mass treatments with antimonials or other agents. However, much of the world's serious disease burden results from so-called anthroponotic leishmaniasis, meaning that humans are the sole major reservoir of the disease-causing parasites.[28,29] Unfortunately, the containment of anthroponotic leishmaniasis generally requires fairly labor-intensive practices such as early diagnosis and treatment and the distribution of insecticide-treated bed nets in order to reduce the likelihood of sandfly bites.[28] Therefore, in many low-income countries where VL occurs, especially in India and Sudan, the lack of access to essential medicines is a major obstacle to control. Among the factors impairing access are the high cost of the medicines, the use of precious hospital beds in order to administer drugs by injection, and the unwillingness of patients to miss time away from work in order to receive their treatments.[28] Access to essential medicines is a particular problem in Bihar State, India, where widespread antimony drug resistance has developed and where more-expensive drugs are required. Some estimates indicate that only 15% of infected patients annually receive treatment in Bihar.[28] In 2005, Bangladesh, India, and Nepal signed an agreement to eliminate VL as a public health problem in the region, although without adequate tools for early diagnosis and options for large-scale treatments, it is not certain at this time whether such efforts will succeed.[28] Clearly, increased access to miltefosine and paromomycin would be of great benefit. Later (in chapter 11), we will explore the possibility of developing an antileishmaniasis vaccine.

Summary Points: the Kinetoplastid Infections

- The kinetoplastid infections are a group of three major human protozoan infections of the poor caused by single-celled parasites with a flagellum and an unusual DNA-containing cell organelle known as the kinetoplastid.
- They frequently occur in areas of conflict or postconflict disruption.

HAT

- HAT, also known as sleeping sickness, occurs annually in an estimated 300,000 to 500,000 people living in sub-Saharan Africa, with the highest rates of infection in war-torn regions of Angola, the DRC, Sudan, and Uganda.
- HAT is caused by two different species of trypanosomes. *T. b. gambiense* is the cause in West Africa, while *T. b. rhodesiense* occurs in East Africa. Both forms are 100% fatal if untreated. Only Uganda has both types of HAT.
- HAT is a vector-transmitted disease, resulting from the bite of tsetses of the genus *Glossina*.
- West African or Gambian HAT is the more chronic form. Parasites circulate in the bloodstream or lymph nodes for years through a process of antigenic variation before the central nervous system phase begins. There are no major animal reservoirs of the disease.
- East African or Rhodesian HAT is the more acute form, and there is a significant animal reservoir. Patients die within one year.
- The drugs used to treat HAT are highly toxic and were developed in the early or middle part of the 20th century.
- Control of West African HAT relies largely on case detection and treatment as well as vector control, while fighting East African HAT relies on control in animal reservoirs and vector control.

Chagas' disease

- Chagas' disease is also known as American trypanosomiasis and is caused by *T. cruzi*. *T. cruzi* has the ability to invade host cells and replicate as amastigotes.
- Approximately 8 to 9 million people are infected with Chagas' disease, all of whom are the poorest people living in the Southern Cone of the Americas, the Andes, the Amazon, or Central America.
- The infection is transmitted by kissing bugs, primarily of the genus *Triatoma* or *Rhodnius*. They often live in the cracks or thatch of low-quality dwellings. Chagas victims often autoinoculate themselves by rubbing contaminated bug feces into their eyes or mouth or through an open wound.
- Acute Chagas' disease is associated with fever, edema, and changes in the conducting system of the heart.

Summary Points *(continued)*

- About 30% of those with acute Chagas' disease will go on to develop the chronic form, associated with cardiomyopathy and megacolon and megaesophagus.
- The efficacy of the two major anti-Chagas' disease drugs is questionable.
- Control of Chagas' disease in the Southern Cone has been highly effective through indoor spraying that targets the vector, *T. infestans*.
- In Central America and elsewhere, control is more problematic.

Leishmaniasis

- Approximately 12 million people are infected with *Leishmania* parasites. In Sudan and elsewhere, highly lethal epidemics of leishmaniasis have occurred over the last 2 decades.
- Leishmaniasis is transmitted by the bite of a sandfly.
- CL is a disfiguring, pizza-like lesion, which often self-heals but can leave a scar. The scar is often deeply stigmatizing for women in developing countries.
- VL, or kala-azar, produces a febrile wasting syndrome with signs and symptoms that resemble leukemia. It can be highly fatal. The greatest numbers of cases of VL are on the Indian subcontinent (India, Nepal, and Bangladesh) and in Sudan and Brazil. VL can also be an opportunistic infection in patients with HIV/AIDS.
- Drugs containing antimony are still widely used for the treatment of CL and VL. However, they are toxic and difficult to administer.
- Because control of VL relies on successful treatment programs, the disease remains widespread in many low-income countries.

chapter 8

The Urban Neglected Tropical Diseases: Leptospirosis, Dengue, and Rabies

If a dog is mad and the authorities have brought the fact to the knowledge of its owner, if he does not keep it in and it bites a man and causes his death, then the owner shall pay two-thirds of a min (40 shekels) of silver. If it bites a slave and causes his death, he shall pay 15 shekels of silver.

ESHMUNA CODE OF BABYLON, 23RD CENTURY BCE

The neglected tropical diseases (NTDs) are infections that primarily occur in regions of rural poverty in developing countries. However, some of the NTDs discussed in the first seven chapters also occur in urban slums and favelas. For instance, ascariasis, one of the unholy trinity of soil-transmitted helminth infections, occurs both in poor urban and rural environments in part because the parasite eggs responsible for transmission are extremely hardy and can sometimes survive in the otherwise unfavorable conditions found in slums. In addition, because some urban-dwelling mosquitoes can transmit *Wuchereria bancrofti* in Africa, India, and elsewhere, lymphatic filariasis (LF) is a problem in some poor urban areas. It has been estimated that almost 30% of people at risk of acquiring LF live in urban settings.[1] Similarly, leishmaniasis, especially the zoonotic form transmitted from dogs, is frequently found in slums.

The NTDs leptospirosis, dengue, and rabies have particular importance as urban health problems in developing countries. For both leptospirosis and dengue, urban flooding is a key component of transmission. As global warming produces an increase in flooding in some regions of the developing world, we can also expect urbanization to combine with climate change to produce an increase in the incidence of these two infections in the coming decades.[2] Also because of climate change, there is a possibility that these NTDs could emerge in urban regions of the United States (discussed in chapter 9).

Leptospirosis

On the edges of Brazil's major urban centers, including Rio de Janeiro, Salvador, and Fortaleza, are crowded slums and shanty towns known as favelas, so named for a plant that thrived in a region where returning Brazilian soldiers once battled against rebel forces in 1897. Upon their return, the soldiers occupied squatters' settlements on the hillsides of Rio de Janeiro. Today, favelas are made up of poor-quality brick and tin-roofed dwellings, usually crowded on the hillsides of Brazil's major cities. They are notorious for their rampant gangs and for frequent drug crimes. Of relevance to the NTDs, the favelas also suffer from frequent floods and do not benefit from regular garbage collection or sewage treatment, thereby creating excellent niches for rats and stray dogs.

It is in this setting of squalor and environmental degradation that the disease leptospirosis finds a welcome home. Leptospirosis is a zoonosis transmitted primarily from rats and dogs. The bacterium that causes leptospirosis (sometimes called a leptospire) is a graceful-looking spiral bacterium that lives for long periods of time in the kidneys of rats and dogs.[3] Leptospires live in association with cells that line the drainage system of the kidneys of these animals. As a result, the urine of rats and dogs living in the favelas teems with millions of leptospires. During certain months of the year when stagnant rainwater collects in the favelas or urban slums (the infection is even found in some slums of inner cities in the United States)[4], the subsequent contamination with rat or dog urine provides a large environmental pool of leptospires and a ready-made mechanism for transmission to humans. Infection typically results when the leptospires penetrate small cuts or abrasions in human skin, such as when favela residents bathe in the canals and other bodies of water. The leptospires also frequently enter through the mucosa of the eyes, nose, and mouth.

Leptospirosis can also occur in rural areas, where leptospires contained in the urine of domestic animals contaminate the soil as well as water.[3] In some developing regions, such as in the Amazon basin, these microbes are also found in a rich diversity of tropical mammals, including bats, rodents, and marsupials.[3] Not surprisingly, people with occupations that require standing in stagnant bodies of water contaminated with animal urine, such as working in sewers and canals, rice and sugarcane harvesting, fish farming, and food processing, are at extremely high risk for the disease.[5] Because leptospires can live in the kidneys of so many different types of mammals, rats are so ubiquitous in urban slums, and transmission is relatively facile, leptospirosis is extremely common in developing countries. Some investigators consider leptospirosis to be the most common zoonosis of humans, although there are few data on the actual prevalence and incidence of this disease.[3] One reason why we know so little about the extent of leptospirosis is that many patients with the infection develop very nonspecific symptoms that can resemble those of other infections.

Following their entry through the skin, the highly motile leptospires have the ability to invade and disseminate to a variety of tissues. Many patients with leptospirosis develop only mild symptoms, while others go on to develop fever, headache, nausea, and vomiting.[3,5] Many of these patients, in turn, have liver involvement as evidenced by jaundice, a condition where the skin turns yellow, similar to viral hepatitis. In about one-fourth of the patients with leptospirosis, this phase is often followed by a second one in which the leptospires invade the central nervous system to produce meningitis,[3] characterized by severe headache and pain behind the eyes. Patients with either the first or second phase of the illness seldom die. However, others can develop a severe form of leptospirosis known as Weil's disease, which is characterized by jaundice, renal failure, and pulmonary hemorrhage (bleeding into the lungs).[3,5] Some patients experience heart involvement. Between 5 and 15% of Weil's disease patients die.[3] Why some patients develop a mild form of the infection versus Weil's disease is not known—it may be related to strain differences of the leptospires, host differences, or a combination of the two factors.

Leptospires are sensitive to many antibiotics in the laboratory, although whether these antibiotics are effective in treating the patient and reducing the severity of the illness is controversial. Many patients have resolution of their illness even if they do not receive antibiotics. Military personnel and travelers to areas where leptospirosis is endemic may benefit from receiving one or more doses of doxycycline as a form of prophylaxis against the illness,[3] but this approach is not practical for widespread use in the favelas. For individuals with high rates of occupational exposure such as sewer workers, wearing protective clothing may help; also, burning sugarcane prior to harvesting diminishes the number of sharp young shoots which can cut the hands and provide a portal of entry for leptospires.[5,6] At the Oswaldo Cruz Foundation in Brazil, efforts are in place to develop a vaccine for leptospirosis. However, until such a vaccine is made readily available, the public health control of leptospirosis relies heavily on having a functioning health system with adequate surveillance for the disease. Adequate surveillance, in turn, usually requires a functional laboratory capable of conducting microbiological diagnosis of leptospirosis through culturing of the organism or through more modern PCR-based assays.[6] Pest (rat) control and local water chlorination are also key features of programs targeting local elimination of leptospirosis.[6] All of these measures require a strong political will on the part of the health ministries in countries where leptospirosis is endemic as well as a highly intact and functional health care system. There is also an urgent need for an international leptospirosis database in order to fully realize the true global burden of this important zoonosis.[7]

Dengue fever (break bone fever)

When the rains fall and surface water collects in canals and sewers, leptospirosis is not the only NTD that the residents of favelas and other urban slums must fear. As water collects in gutters, cisterns, and other water storage

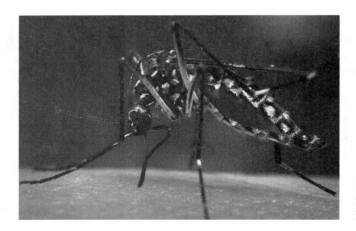

Figure 8.1 A. *aegypti*, the mosquito vector of dengue fever (Public Health Image Library, CDC [http://phil.cdc.gov]).

containers and even in discarded tires, it creates a breeding ground for mosquitoes. Among the major mosquitoes that breed in this environment are *Anopheles* mosquitoes, which can transmit LF and malaria, as well as the *Aedes* mosquitoes, especially *Aedes aegypti* (Fig. 8.1), which transmit the flaviviruses that cause dengue fever and yellow fever.

Through aggressive vector control efforts in South America during the 1960s, the urban foci of both yellow fever and dengue fever began to diminish, so that by the late 1960s these infections had almost been eradicated in the tropical regions of the continent.[8,9] However, with the subsequent suspension of many of these programs during the 1970s, *Aedes* mosquito breeding resumed. By the middle 1990s, maps showing the geographic distribution of this insect vector resembled vector maps made 30 years earlier.[9] This situation is not too different from the reemergence of human African trypanosomiasis in Angola, the Democratic Republic of the Congo, and Sudan, which resulted from interruption of tsetse control efforts, but in the case of South America it was a voluntary suspension of vector control rather than one that was forced by conflict. Today in Brazil, it has been estimated that every year there are thousands of cases of dengue fever, most of them in the favelas of the hot and tropical northeastern regions.[8] In such Brazilian favelas, epidemics occur in May through July, a period that follows the heaviest rains by approximately 2 to 3 months. This period corresponds to that required for several life cycles of the *Aedes* vector to build up and transmit dengue fever on a community-wide scale.[8] According to the World Health Organization, in 2001, more than 600,000 cases were reported from the Americas.[10]

Dengue fever is distributed throughout the poor urban areas of the tropics. The global prevalence of dengue is unknown, although there may be as many as 50 million people infected annually, making this NTD the most frequent arboviral infection (arthropod-borne viral infection) worldwide.[10] Dengue is also one of the most serious consequences of increasing urbanization in the developing world. As human populations continue to migrate from rural areas to the cities, the ever-expanding slums, shantytowns, and favelas provide ideal ecological niches for *Aedes* mosquitoes.[8] Such migrations, together with flooding that can result from global warming, largely account for the estimated 30-fold increase in dengue outbreaks over the last 50 years.[11] In the Americas, the first dengue outbreaks occurred in Cuba in 1977–1978, followed by subsequent outbreaks there in 1981 and 1997, as well as outbreaks in Venezuela.[7] In all, more than 30 Latin American countries have reported dengue outbreaks.[11] Because *Aedes* mosquitoes also thrive in Florida and other parts of the American South, it would not be too surprising if outbreaks appeared among the poor living in the slums of urban centers along the Gulf Coast, including New Orleans. Today, the largest number of cases of dengue fever occur in Asia, particularly Southeast Asia, India and Sri Lanka, southern China (especially Hainan Province), and the South Pacific islands (especially Fiji).[11] Dengue fever is also common in coastal regions of sub-Saharan Africa.

The virus that causes dengue fever belongs to a family of flaviviruses, which also comprise other tropical pathogens, including the viruses that cause yellow fever, West Nile fever, and Japanese encephalitis. A characteristic feature of the flaviviruses is that their genome is comprised of a single strand of RNA, as opposed to our human double-stranded DNA genome.[11] Another important feature is that there are four antigenically distinct types (called serotypes) of dengue viruses.[11] This observation will become relevant when we discuss some of the severe complications that can result from dengue infection. Dengue virus replicates in the salivary glands of *Aedes* mosquitoes. *A. aegypti* is the major but not the only species of the *Aedes* genus. *A. aegypti* usually bites during the day. After humans become infected, the virus migrates to the lymph nodes and then to the bloodstream, where the virus disseminates widely throughout the body.[12] Infants and young children, when they become infected for the first time, often develop an illness characterized by high fever which is difficult to distinguish from other common childhood illnesses. However, older children and adults often develop classical dengue fever, often known as break bone fever, so named because of the high fever accompanied by headache and severe muscle, joint, and bone pain.[12] Flushing is also commonly observed on the face, neck, and chest.

The most dreaded complication is dengue hemorrhagic fever (DHF),[11] which typically occurs in children (less than 16 years of age) who experience two sequential dengue infections of two different serotypes within an interval of several years.[12] The mechanism by which DHF occurs in children with two different serotypes of dengue is not known, although it has been hypothesized by Scott Halstead (formerly of the Rockefeller Foundation and now with the Pediatric Dengue Vaccine Initiative) and others that the host immune response is somehow involved.[13] The major clinical features of DHF include high fever for several days, with hemorrhagic complications, especially bleeding from the gut, gums, and vagina, and a drop in the number of platelets circulating in the bloodstream.[11] Some patients with DHF progress to liver failure and dengue shock syndrome, which is associated with circulatory collapse and profound shock. The mortality rate of shock syndrome can approach 50% and accounts for a large percentage of the estimated several thousand deaths from dengue that occur every year.[11] Epidemics of DHF are dramatic because they primarily target large numbers of children and present with profoundly disturbing hemorrhagic complications. During outbreaks, it is not uncommon to have entire pediatric wards filled with crying and bleeding children. The number of DHF outbreaks is on the rise in Asia; the first epidemic was reported from Manila in 1954 and was succeeded by a severe and noteworthy rise in epidemics beginning in 1980, including those in Indonesia, Vietnam, Sri Lanka, Hainan Province (China), and Fiji.[11] In these regions, overall dengue transmission is high and there are at least two different dengue serotypes appearing in an interval of a few years. In the Americas, DHF outbreaks have occurred recently in more than 20 countries.[11] The Cuban DHF epidemic in 1981 resulted from a type 2 dengue virus imported from Southeast Asia and occurred four years following a type 1 dengue epidemic in 1977.[11,12] In 2001 the World Health Assembly passed a resolution advocating increased global surveillance efforts. In response, the World Health Organization established DengueNET in order to increase the efficiency of global monitoring efforts.[14]

Ultimately, the long-term control of dengue fever and DHF will require the development of a safe and effective vaccine. Later (in chapter 11), we will discuss ongoing international efforts to do precisely that. In the meantime, our current approach to dengue control relies on a rather labor-intensive, aggressive, and multidisciplinary approach comprising environmental control methods to reduce the number of available vector breeding sites (through rigorous drainage or destruction of open vessels containing rainwater), insecticidal spraying, and improvements in house design.[11] For instance, during periods of dengue outbreaks in Singapore, the National Environmental Agency employs 500 inspectors who conduct house-to-house searches in any area where two cases of dengue occur within 14 days of each other and within a 150-m radius.[15] In such areas, the inspectors check for standing bodies of water in gutters, in potted plants, or between the leaves of palm trees.[15] Such methods were partly responsible for the reduction of malaria, yellow fever, and other vector-borne diseases that allowed construction of the Panama Canal during the early 20th century. Unfortunately, many developing countries cannot afford a sophisticated public health infrastructure like the one presently in place in Singapore. Until a vaccine becomes available, however, there are not many alternatives to house-to-house mosquito "search and destroy" missions. In contrast to malaria and LF control efforts in which insecticide-treated bed nets have a role in interrupting transmission by night-biting *Anopheles* mosquitoes, this approach has not been of much value for the day-biting *A. aegypti* mosquito.[11] In some dengue-plagued regions, such as in Vietnam, biological control with copepod crustaceans and other agents[16] has also met with some success.

Rabies

Of all the infections plaguing humankind, rabies is among the most terrifying. Once contracted and once clinical signs become evident, rabies is almost invariably fatal. Most patients die a truly horrible death by first developing a condition known as furious rabies, the hallmark of which is hydrophobia (fear of water).[17] In hydrophobia, an effort to drink water, or in some cases even the sound of water or the thought of water, provokes a reflex contraction of the throat and diaphragm (as well as of other muscles of inspiratory respiration) accompanied by expressions of abject fear and terror.[17] This condition lasts for about 1 week before coma and paralysis take over prior to death.

The dramatic end game of rabies and the fear that it generated are no doubt responsible for why we can find unambiguous descriptions of rabies in texts from ancient Egypt, Greece, Rome, and China.[18] There is even a reference to rabies in the Babylon Codex, 23 centuries BCE, a quotation from which is provided at the beginning of this chapter.[18] Today, human rabies is mostly an urban disease found in developing countries. While sporadic cases of human rabies transmitted from bats (and, rarely, from skunks and raccoons) occur in the United States and elsewhere in the industrialized world, most of the 55,000 people who contract rabies and die annually live in Asia and Africa, where the infection is endemic in dogs.[19] In India, where more than half of the annual rabies deaths occur (about 30,000 cases), approximately 96% of the cases are contracted through dog bites.[20] Most of the deaths in India occur among very poor adult males.[20] In the vast majority of the cases both in India and elsewhere, urban rabies is transmitted by the bite of a stray dog. It is estimated that India has a dog population of about 25 million, most of which are ownerless.[20]

Almost as serious as its enormous toll on human life is the economic impact of rabies.[21] In the United States, pet owners spend an estimated $300 million annually to vaccinate their pet dogs and cats, while in developing countries, there are enormous costs associated with administering rabies vaccine to individuals bitten by dogs.[19,21] After someone is bitten by a rabid dog, one of the few opportunities to reduce the odds of developing clinical rabies (and dying) is to receive a rabies vaccine through what is known as postexposure prophylaxis (PEP). The fear and anxiety of developing rabies, and the potentially horrific outcome if no vaccine is given, mean that for every fatal case of rabies, thousands more receive PEP annually. For instance, in Thailand more than 100,000 people receive PEP every year at a cost of US$10 million,[21] while throughout Asia, an estimated 7 million people receive PEP. The highest rate of PEP administration occurs in Vietnam.[22]

Following a bite by a rabid animal, saliva containing the rabies virus is introduced into the skin and muscle, where the virus replicates before it attaches to neuronal cell membranes by specific receptors.[23] If a bite victim does not receive PEP, the rabies virus then travels retrograde along peripheral nerves at a rate of approximately 5 to 10 cm (2 to 5 in.) per day, until it reaches the central nervous system.[23] Once the rabies virus reaches the central nervous system, the patient's fate is sealed. Exactly how the rabies virus causes such severe disease in the brain, especially in a part of the brain known as the limbic system, as suggested by the clinical picture of furious rabies, is not well known. Among the hypotheses under investigation are that the virus somehow disrupts neuronal metabolism or causes formation of interneuronal connections.[23] Conceivably, a better understanding of this process could lead to new and innovative interventions for people who already show clinical signs of the disease.

The first rabies vaccine was developed by Louis Pasteur in the 19th century. This development led to the establishment of Pasteur Institutes all over the Francophone world, which made available first-generation rabies vaccine to many developing countries. Since then, the process of developing rabies vaccine has been refined such that modern rabies vaccine production now uses in vitro cell culture methods for growing the vaccine strain of the virus rather than Pasteur's original method of using neural tissues from animals. The toxicities and side effects of the older, neural tissue-derived vaccines make them highly undesirable, and there are even concerns that some of the vaccines are not very effective. However, even after a century, high-quality, cell culture-derived rabies vaccine is still not widely available in developing countries. For instance, a sheep brain-derived vaccine known as Semple is produced in the Indian subcontinent, and suckling mouse-brain vaccine is made in Vietnam, Africa, and South America.[23] Global efforts to transfer the technology for cell culture-derived rabies vaccine to India and elsewhere in developing countries are in progress. In addition to developing human vaccines for PEP, there is also a need to increase rates of vaccination of stray dogs in the urban centers of developing countries. For instance, mass vaccination campaigns have resulted in the elimination of rabies from Japan and Taiwan and many urban areas in South America.[17] There is an urgent need to vaccinate stray dogs throughout the urban centers of India, Bangladesh, and wherever the number of annual rabies deaths is high.

Summary

According to the UN Population Fund, now, for the first time, more than half (3.3 billion people) of the world's population is living in cities and towns, and by 2030, almost 5 billion people will live in urban areas.[1,24] Increasing urbanization is expected to bring with it serious increases in urban poverty, and the slums, favelas, and shantytowns are expected only to get worse. Today almost 1 billion people live in slums, i.e., approximately 32% of the global urban population and 43% of the world's developing-country population (see report summary at http://www.unhabitat.org).[25] Unless significant steps are taken to reduce squalor in the urban areas of the developing world, we can anticipate increases in dengue, leptospirosis, rabies, and other urban NTDs. The UN Population Fund asserts that, as our world's cities expand, we need to embrace the concepts of respecting the rights of the poor and promoting access to clean water, waste disposal, and power.[24] Otherwise, we risk condemning the next urban generation to a life of poverty and misery.

Summary Points: the Urban NTDs

- Leptospirosis, dengue fever, and rabies are important NTDs found in the urban slums and favelas of developing countries.
- Today, approximately one-half of the world's population lives in urban areas.

Leptospirosis

- Leptospirosis is one of the world's most common zoonoses, transmitted through contact with bodies of water, e.g., canals and sewers, contaminated with leptospires.
- In urban areas, contamination occurs through exposure to the urine of rats and stray dogs, which teems with leptospires.
- Many patients with leptospirosis develop a nonspecific febrile illness or aseptic meningitis. The most severe complication is Weil's disease, which has a high mortality rate.
- Adequate prevention requires having an intact system of surveillance and case detection as well as environmental control.

Dengue fever

- Dengue fever is one of the most common NTDs of urban areas, with an estimated 50 million cases worldwide. The number of dengue cases, possibly more than that of any other NTD, is expected to continue to rise as a consequence of increasing urbanization and global warming.
- Dengue is caused by a single-stranded RNA flavivirus and transmitted by the bite of a female *Aedes* mosquito. *A. aegypti* is the most common insect vector species.
- Like leptospirosis, most dengue cases present as a nonspecific febrile illness. However, classical dengue is sometimes known as break bone fever because of the severe myalgias and headache that can accompany the illness.
- The most feared complication of dengue is DHF, which is associated with severe morbidity. DHF occurs as a result of infection with two different serotypes of the dengue virus separated by a period of years. Some patients with DHF will die from dengue shock syndrome.
- No vaccine is yet available for dengue. Presently public health control relies on labor-intensive practices of environmental vector control.
- A WHO-based global surveillance network, DengueNET, is in place.

Rabies

- Rabies has been one of the most feared infections since ancient times.
- Approximately 50,000 people die from rabies annually. Most of these deaths occur as the result of stray-dog bites in developing countries. More than half of the cases occur in India alone.

Summary Points *(continued)*

- There is also an enormous economic toll from rabies. This is because of the need to administer PEP with rabies vaccine to almost anyone bitten by a dog in developing countries.
- Many developing-country manufacturers still produce rabies vaccines derived from neural tissues. Such vaccines may have associated toxicities and are often not as effective as newer-generation vaccines that use in vitro cell culture methods.
- The public health control of rabies in many countries has been achieved through aggressive campaigns to vaccinate dogs in urban centers.

chapter 9

The Neglected Tropical Diseases of North America

A civilization is judged by the treatment of its minorities.

Mahatma Gandhi

Although the NTDs are not as prominent in the United States, Canada, Mexico, and the Caribbean as they are in the low-income countries of Africa, Asia, and Central and South America, these infections are nonetheless significant among the poorest people living in North America. Many of the North American NTDs are also zoonoses, meaning that they are transmitted from animals to people. Populations at particular risk for acquiring these NTDs include minority populations such as African-Americans and Hispanics, as well as many of North America's Native Americans. A serious NTD problem resulting from endemic hookworm infection, lymphatic filariasis (LF), and schistosomiasis also occurs in the Caribbean region, where it has been argued that these diseases represent a glaring legacy of the Atlantic slave trade. Today, the persistence of the NTDs in North America, considered one of the world's wealthiest continents, represents a health disparity of astonishing proportions.

NTDs in the United States

Historically, the most impoverished populations living in the United States have suffered greatly from NTDs. In many respects the rural American South at the beginning of the 20th century resembled a developing country, with high rates of hookworm infection and other soil-transmitted helminthiases, as well as endemic malaria, pellagra (a nutritional deficiency of nicotinic acid), typhoid fever, and seasonal epidemics of yellow fever.[1] Indeed, the pejorative concept of the "lazy Southerner" was partly a consequence of the toxic combination of chronic parasitism and nutritional deficiencies that plagued this region, as the NTDs kept the southern population mired in poverty just as they do today in Africa, Asia, and elsewhere. The medical historian Margaret Humphreys has argued effectively that New Deal programs (including the Agricultural Adjustment Act) during the 1930s did more than anything else to reduce the burden of tropical diseases in the United States by relocating agricultural workers to urban areas and transforming the American South from an agrarian economy into an urbanized, industrial one.[1] It is still true that urbanization and parallel economic development are the most potent forces in melting away the NTDs, just as they were in Japan and Korea after World War II and in China beginning in the 1990s.

Today, as a result of dramatic economic gains, tropical afflictions such as malaria, pellagra, and typhoid fever are no longer endemic in the United States. However, several NTDs still remain among our nation's poorest people. According to the U.S. Census, our nation's official poverty rate stands at 12.3%, with approximately 36.5 million Americans living in poverty.[2] However, among African-American and Hispanic populations, the poverty rate exceeds 20%. At a poverty rate of 17.4%, children also suffer disproportionately from poverty.[2] Of the 36.5 million impoverished Americans, the Poverty in America Project (http://povertyinamerica.psu.edu) estimates that 15.9 million Americans live in "abject poverty," meaning that they make a bare-bones sum of US$437 per month with no more than US$50 per week available for food.[2] Some of these impoverished Americans are at risk for several NTDs discussed previously in this book, including the soil-transmitted helminth infections, trachoma, Chagas' disease, leishmaniasis, and two of the major urban NTDs, leptospirosis and dengue fever. They are also at risk for two zoonotic NTDs not discussed previously, namely, cysticercosis and toxoplasmosis.

The soil-transmitted helminth infections (toxocariasis and strongyloidiasis)

Prominent among the American NTDs are the soil-transmitted helminth infections. When last studied during the 1960s and 1970s, pockets of hookworm infection, as well as ascariasis and trichuriasis, still occurred among the rural poor living in regions where those diseases had been highly endemic, especially southeastern Georgia, the Gulf Coast regions of southern Mississippi, the coastal Carolinas, and East Texas near the Sabine River.[3] At one time, the Eastern Cherokees stood out as a population with particularly high rates of infection.[4] While hookworm is probably no longer a serious public health threat in the rural American South, we do not know for sure, since large-scale epidemiological studies of hookworm infection and other soil-transmitted helminth infections in the United States have not been conducted within the last 3 decades. Therefore, it is important to revisit some of the vulnerable populations living in this part of the United States and reassess the prevalence of the unholy trinity in their communities.

Today, we know that at least two soil-transmitted helminth infections are still significant diseases in the United States—toxocariasis and strongyloidiasis. Toxocariasis is a zoonosis that results when humans accidentally ingest the eggs of a dog ascarid parasite known as *Toxocara canis*. A high percentage of puppies are infected with *Toxocara* worms, which in many respects are equivalent to the canine counterpart of the human soil-transmitted helminth *Ascaris lumbricoides*. Because puppies indiscriminately defecate on the ground, particularly in urban areas of the United States as well as in some rural areas, *T. canis* and other ascarid eggs are extremely common in the environment. For instance, in Wallingford, CT, a small city located halfway between Hartford and New Haven, 27.5% of public playground areas were found to be contaminated with *Toxocara* eggs.[5] Probably more than any other group, children from poor families come into contact with these eggs as a result of exposure to the feces of *Toxocara*-infected stray dogs defecating on dirt and sandy areas of inner-city playgrounds. When children accidentally ingest the eggs, the eggs hatch and the released *T. canis* larvae migrate through the major organs of the body (Fig. 9.1). By so doing, *T. canis* larvae cause a serious syndrome of toddlers known as visceral larval migrans, which is characterized by fever and inflammation in the liver (hepatitis) and lungs (pneumonitis). Visceral larva migrans is also often accompanied by allergic symptoms, including wheezing (Fig. 9.1). A second syndrome resulting from *Toxocara* infection, known as ocular larva migrans, also occurs in older children, in which *T. canis* larvae migrate to the eye, where they cause retinitis and strabismus. Many children also acquire a third form of *Toxocara* infection known as covert toxocariasis. Covert toxocariasis is characterized by eosinophilia, i.e., an increase in a type of white blood cell known as the eosinophil, as well as wheezing and other symptoms that resemble asthma.[6] Because *T. canis* can sometimes migrate through the brain, it is believed that toxocariasis may be linked to neuropsychiatric disturbances.

Unfortunately, there are very few studies to document the extent of any of these three forms of toxocariasis in the United States. During the 1970s, it was determined that between 4.6 and 7.3% of children in different geographic regions of the United States were found to have some form of *T. canis* infection. However, among African-American children with lower socioeconomic status, up to 30% were infected.[7] Later, in the 1990s, a team led by myself and Neda Sharghi, then a Yale University graduate public health student, conducted studies among children in some of Connecticut's poor urban areas (New Haven and Bridgeport) and found that 10% of these inner-city children showed evidence of infection at some point in their lives, as evidenced by having measurable antibody to *T. canis*.[8] Among poor Hispanic children living in Bridgeport, up to 50% showed evidence of previous infection.[8] An earlier study in New York City found that 5% of blood samples from children which were submitted for lead testing were also positive for previous *T. canis* infection.[9] The relationship between toxocariasis and lead ingestion may be more than coincidental, since

Toxocariasis
(Toxocara canis, Toxocara cati)

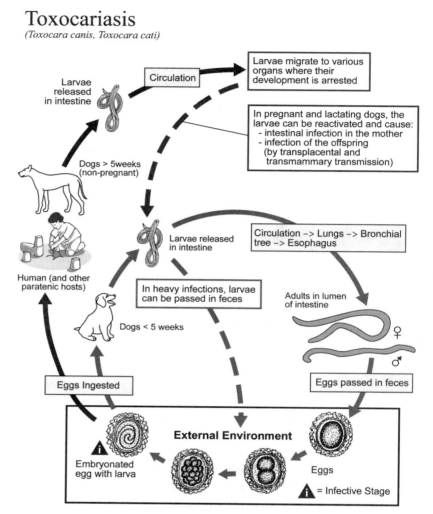

Figure 9.1 The life cycle of human infection with *T. canis* (Public Health Image Library, CDC [http://phil.cdc.gov]).

the same behavior responsible for ingesting lead paint chips might also pro-mote ingestion of substances contaminated with egg-containing dirt.

Children living in inner cities have a higher frequency and severity of asthma attacks than do other pediatric populations living in the United States.[10] Could covert toxocariasis account for a portion of our nation's asthma epidemic? We were not able to show this relationship conclusively in Connecticut, although studies in Europe and elsewhere have demonstrated an important link between *Toxocara* infection and asthma.[11] Given that 5% or more of inner-city children in the Northeast may have had *Toxocara* infection at some point during their lives, we are likely looking at a large number of U.S. children at risk for covert toxocariasis. For instance, if we look at the combined African-American and Hispanic populations of our major East Coast cities and assume a 5% infection rate among these populations, then possibly up to 323,000 people have had past exposure to *T. canis* infection.[12] If we include major Southern cities such as Atlanta, Houston, and Miami, this number increases to 500,000. Thus, there is a possibility that a half-million inner-city American children either have or had toxocariasis. Because this infection may place these children at risk for asthma and other illnesses, such information suggests an urgent need to conduct larger and better surveillance studies for this illness among U.S. inner-city children.

Still another potentially important soil-transmitted helminth infection in the United States is strongyloidiasis, a severe cause of enteritis (inflammation of the intestine) with diarrhea. Strongyloidiasis is also a potentially fatal disseminated infection in patients who are immunocompromised from receiving steroids. Worldwide, approximately 30 million or more people are infected with *Strongyloides stercoralis*, primarily in rural, developing regions of Asia, Africa, and the Americas. However, strongyloidiasis has also been shown to be endemic in the rural Appalachian region of the United States. Although our existing data are severely limited, studies conducted over the past few decades have shown that the prevalence of endemic strongyloidiasis in the rural counties of eastern Kentucky and Tennessee ranges from 1 to 4%.[13] Overall, the population of rural Appalachia is approximately 6.8 million.[14] If we estimate that 1% of this population is infected with strongyloidiasis, then there are approximately 68,000 cases of strongyloidiasis in the region. Again, it is important to fully explore the extent of this disease in the United States.

Cysticercosis and neurocysticercosis

Cysticercosis is an NTD that results in seizures and other long-term neurological manifestations. It results from transmission from person to person of the eggs of the pork tapeworm, *Taenia solium*. The life cycle of *T. solium* infection is shown in Fig. 9.2. Humans acquire the pork tapeworm by ingesting the cyst stages of the parasite, known as cysticerci, which are found in the muscles and brains of infected pigs. Following ingestion of these cysts as a result of eating uncooked or improperly cooked pork, an immature larva will fasten onto the intestinal wall and begin growing into an adult tapeworm. The adult pork tapeworm can reach huge lengths in the human gut, often 2 or 3 m, but having a huge tapeworm surprisingly causes very little in the way of symptoms. When a person harbors a pork tapeworm, however, segments of the parasite containing eggs can break off in the intestine. These egg-sac-like segments exit the body in feces. When pigs ingest fecal material containing eggs (in some very poor regions, it is a common practice to feed human feces to pigs), the eggs hatch and give rise to cysticerci in the muscles or brains of the animal.

Cysticercosis is the more serious condition resulting from *T. solium* infection and occurs when humans accidentally ingest *T. solium* eggs excreted by a household member (often a person from a country such as Mexico or El Salvador where cysticercosis is endemic) who is infected with the adult tapeworm. An infected person can sometimes shed thousands of eggs daily, and the transmission of the eggs from one person to another (typically through accidental fecal-oral contamination) gives rise to this condition. After the eggs

Cysticercosis

(Taenia spp.)

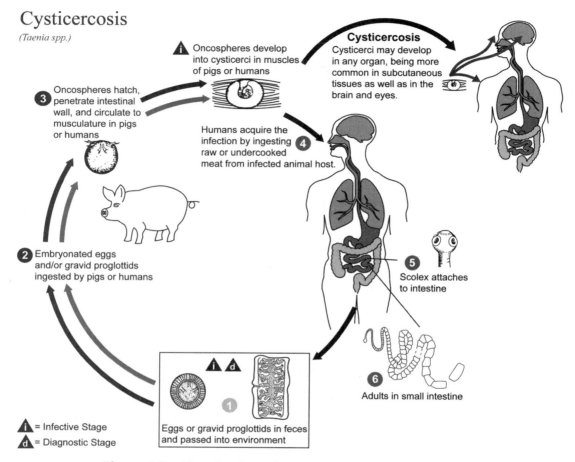

Figure 9.2 Life cycle of *T. solium* and cysticercosis (Public Health Image Library, CDC [http://phil.cdc.gov]).

are swallowed, larvae known as oncospheres are liberated; these invade the gut wall and enter the human circulatory system. The larvae travel to the muscles and brain, where they form cysts. In the muscles, *T. solium* infection usually does not cause much in the way of symptoms, but the presence of *T. solium* cysts in the brain can trigger severe and unremitting seizures unless the patient is treated immediately with anticonvulsant medication. In some cases, multiple cysts can cause more extensive disease such as encephalitis, while cysts at the base of the brain can cause obstruction of the flow of cerebrospinal fluid, leading to a condition known as hydrocephalus. The diagnosis of cysticercosis in the brain (sometimes known as neurocysticercosis) usually requires special radiographic imaging with either computerized axial tomography or magnetic resonance imaging, while treatment requires use of anticonvulsants and sometimes anthelmintic drugs such as albendazole and praziquantel.

    In part because of the large influx of Hispanic migrants from Mexico to the United States, as well as the arrival of Central American immigrants (there are an estimated 20 million Mexicans and almost 2 million Central American immigrants living in the United States), neurocysticercosis has become a serious infection in Texas, New Mexico, Arizona, and California, as well as in Chicago and New York.[15] Across the country, children and adults are today being brought into emergency rooms with seizures and being diagnosed with neurocysticercosis. Over the last 20 years, almost 1,500 cases of neurocysticercosis have been reported, but it has been only within the last few years that many states have mandated reporting at all. Today an estimated 1,000 to 2,000 new cases of neurocysticercosis are diagnosed annually,[16] making it one of the leading causes of epilepsy in the United States. However, at an incidence of 8 to 10 per 100,000 per year among Hispanic populations,[17] and considering that there are approximately 35 million Hispanics living in the United States, as many as 2,800 to 3,500 new cases of cysticercosis may occur annually. In a study conducted in rural Ventura County, CA, it was determined that 1.8% of that population had antibodies to the *Taenia* parasites that cause cysticercosis.[18] If we use this value and extrapolate for the entire rural Hispanic population of the United States (estimated at 2.3 million in 2000 [http://factfinder.census.gov]), then it is conceivable that the number of people living with cysticercosis in the United States may be much higher, possibly as many as 41,400. Not surprisingly, neurocysticercosis now accounts for 10% of neurology and neurosurgery admissions and 10% of all seizures presenting to some emergency rooms in Los Angeles.[18] Presumably, this is the experience of other large Southwestern U.S. cities with large Hispanic populations. The large number of possible cases of cysticercosis suggests that there is an urgent need for better surveillance studies on the presence of this condition in the Southwestern United States and for treatment of patients who harbor the pork tapeworm as a means of reducing the prevalence of this serious disease of poverty.

Toxoplasmosis and giardiasis

One of the most serious protozoan infections occurring in the United States is toxoplasmosis. Caused by *Toxoplasma gondii*, it has two major routes of infection, either ingestion of a form of the parasite found in cat feces known as the oocyst (which may occur when changing kitty litter) or ingestion of uncooked meat (primarily pork) contaminated with the bradyzoite stages of the parasite (Fig. 9.3). Roughly one-half of the cases occur by either route. Toxoplasmosis is very common in the United States—approximately 15% of U.S. residents have antibodies to *T. gondii*, meaning that they have been infected with these parasites. However, Mexican-Americans and African-Americans have a higher rate of infection.[19]

Most people who become infected with toxoplasmosis do not become very ill. Often, this infection is a nonspecific illness accompanied by fever and swelling of the lymph nodes. It is therefore easy to confuse toxoplasmosis with other infectious illnesses, especially many viral infections. However, one population is particularly vulnerable to severe effects of *T. gondii* infection, namely, the unborn fetus. If a pregnant mother becomes infected with *T. gondii* during her pregnancy, especially early in the pregnancy, the newborn infant can be born

Toxoplasmosis
(Toxoplasma gondii)

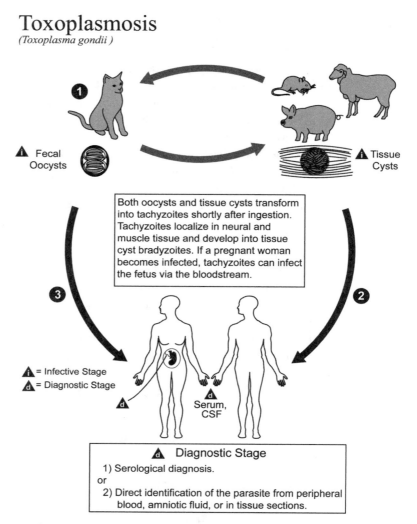

Figure 9.3 Life cycle of *T. gondii* (Public Health Image Library, CDC [http://phil.cdc.gov]). CSF, cerebrospinal fluid.

with congenital toxoplasmosis, a syndrome that includes vision impairment and blindness, hearing loss, seizures, and mental retardation. The Centers for Disease Control and Prevention (CDC) estimates that of the 4 million live infants born each year in the United States, approximately 400 to 4,000 have congenital toxoplasmosis.[20] The National Collaborative Chicago-Based, Congenital Toxoplasmosis Study has recently concluded a 20-year study of 120 infants with congenital toxoplasmosis and found that early diagnosis and treatment for a year with antiparasitic drugs can make a huge difference in the long-term clinical outcomes of these children.[21] However, many infants do not show obvious evidence of congenital toxoplasmosis at birth. Instead, the disease is not overtly manifested until later in the 1st year, and by then treatment may be too late to prevent the most serious consequences of the infection. Beginning in 1986, the Commonwealth of Massachusetts began conducting universal screening of newborns, a program similar to the screening for phenylketonuria and other genetic disorders. Over the last 20 years, an estimated 50 cases of congenital toxoplasmosis have been detected and treated.[22] Sadly, only New Hampshire has joined Massachusetts in conducting newborn screening through a New England Newborn Screening Program. It is essential to conduct nationwide newborn screening in order to identify the thousands of infants born every year with congenital toxoplasmosis. We will see below that toxoplasmosis is also an important public health threat among the Inuit of the Canadian Arctic, making them a population also worth screening.

Giardiasis is an intestinal protozoan infection occurring commonly in the United States. It results from the ingestion of *Giardia intestinalis* cysts contained in contaminated water or food. Transmitted by the fecal-oral route, *Giardia* infection is considered a major cause of diarrhea in day care centers.[23] It is also found in public bathing areas and occasionally contaminates drinking water. The proportion of cases resulting from waterborne outbreaks versus day care center outbreaks versus other modes of transmission is not known. Many patients who acquire giardiasis never develop any symptoms. However, a significant number of infected people develop acute diarrhea and some children experience a syndrome characterized by chronic diarrhea, fat malabsorption, and weight loss. Giardiasis is an extremely common infection worldwide, and in the United States the CDC estimates that between 424,120 and 2,120,600 cases (147.3 to 736.4 cases per 100,000) occur,[23] although no data exist on whether the proportion of cases is higher among socioeconomically disadvantaged groups.

Leishmaniasis and Chagas' disease

Earlier (in chapter 7), information on the persistence of cutaneous leishmaniasis (CL) in the Americas was presented. Dozens of cases of CL have now been reported from south-central Texas, suggesting that this condition may be becoming an important NTD in the region.[24] In 2007, nine cases of CL were also detected in north Texas. Indigenous CL in Texas is caused by *Leishmania mexicana*, and it is believed that wood-burrowing rats may serve as reservoir hosts. CL has also been identified as an important NTD among the U.S. troops returning from Operation Iraqi Freedom.[24] Visceral leishmaniasis (VL) has been documented from dogs in the United States, especially foxhounds. There is a potential for transmission of VL to humans to become a serious public health problem in the United States.[24] Similarly, it has been estimated that as many as 150,000 Latin American immigrants living in the United States may develop chronic Chagas' disease, and there is a serious risk of transmission because kissing bug vectors are found in the American South.[24]

Trachoma

Earlier (in chapter 5), we discussed trachoma as an important infectious cause of blindness in developing countries, particularly in dry and dusty areas of the Sahel. Over the last few decades in the American Southwest, trachoma has been a well-known public health problem among the Navajo Indians living on the Navajo Reservation.[25]

Dengue and leptospirosis

As discussed earlier (in chapter 8), the major urban NTDs include leptospirosis, dengue, and rabies. Today, both dengue and leptospirosis occur sporadically in the United States, but we can expect that the number of cases will increase in the coming decade. For dengue, 62,514 cases were reported in the three Mexican states bordering Texas between 1980 and 1999, and presently *Aedes* mosquitoes are found throughout the American South.[26] Dengue transmission also occurs commonly in Puerto Rico.[26] Similarly, leptospirosis is found in slum areas of major urban centers, including Baltimore and Detroit, and is also found frequently in Hawaii.[26] With the increased flooding that may result from global warming and other climate changes, we should anticipate that both dengue and leptospirosis could become increasing problems in the United States.[26]

NTDs in Arctic Canada and Alaska

The Inuit are a group of approximately 150,000 indigenous people inhabiting the Arctic regions of Canada (including Nunavut, northern Quebec and Labrador, and the Northwest Territories), Alaska, and Greenland, where, for most of their history, they have pursued a largely nomadic lifestyle, with a heavy reliance on hunting and fishing. Over the last few decades, most of the Inuit have relocated to permanent settlements. There they face enormous challenges, including overcrowding, high rates of poverty and unemployment, alcoholism and other substance abuse, depression, and suicide. In the absence of fresh vegetables and fruit in the Arctic tundra and taiga areas, the diet of the Inuit relies heavily on meat, especially from sea mammals and polar bear. Such a diet makes them vulnerable to at least two major food-borne parasitic diseases: trichinellosis (also known as trichinosis) and toxoplasmosis. In addition, the close association between the Inuit and sled dogs, reindeer, and elk makes them susceptible to another NTD known as echinococcosis.

Trichinellosis (trichinosis)

Like toxoplasmosis and pork tapeworm infection, trichinellosis is commonly acquired through the ingestion of uncooked pork. The newborn larval stages of *Trichinella spiralis spiralis* (*T. s. spiralis*), a nematode parasite, typically live in the flesh of pigs, and outbreaks of the disease occurred throughout the continental United States during the 20th century. Such outbreaks were caused partly by the appalling conditions in U.S. slaughterhouses, which included the practice of allowing pigs to feed on infected rats and uncooked garbage. Such practices were described by Upton Sinclair in his depictions of meat packing plants in his early-20th-century novel *The Jungle*. Trichinellosis begins as a disease that resembles an attack of food poisoning with nausea and vomiting, usually occurring within a week after ingestion of *Trichinella*-contaminated meat. This so-called enteric phase is followed by the muscle or invasion phase, characterized by severe muscle pain as well as edema around the eyelids (periorbital edema) and eosinophilia. Death can result from large infestations in the muscle or when *Trichinella* larvae invade the heart muscle.

Trichinellosis caused by *T. s. spiralis* is no longer a significant public health problem in the United States, but a variant of the disease caused by *T. s. nativa* is now an important problem among the Inuit. For instance, multiple outbreaks have occurred in Nunavik (the Inuit region in northern Quebec) over the past few decades.[27] Trichinellosis caused by *T. s. nativa* produces a syndrome similar to *T. s. spiralis* infection, but repeated infections cause primarily intestinal symptoms, including prolonged diarrhea, rather than severe muscle pain.[28] Most of the Canadian Arctic trichinellosis outbreaks result from raw or insufficiently cooked walrus meat, although other outbreaks have resulted from the consumption of foxes and polar bears. An estimated 60% of polar bears are infected with *Trichinella* larvae, while only 2 to 4% of walruses are infected.[27,28] Interestingly, *T. s. spiralis*, the major species of *Trichinella* parasites that caused disease in the 20th-century United States, is susceptible to destruction both through heat (cooking) and prolonged freezing. However, *T. s. nativa*, the major Arctic *Trichinella* species found in polar bears and walruses, has specifically adapted through evolution to resist freezing.[27,28] In Nunavik, an innovative prevention program (developed by J. Dick MacLean and his colleagues at the McGill University Centre for Tropical Diseases at the Montreal General Hospital together with Jean-François Proulx from the Nunavik Regional Board of Health and Social Services) has been established in which preconsumption testing of tagged samples from walrus is conducted at a regional laboratory.[27,28] Any urgent information is communicated immediately to the local community by radio in order to ensure that no infected meat is consumed. Those who had infected meat are treated prophylactically with the anthelmintic drug mebendazole in order to abort the trichinellosis infection and prevent larvae from entering the muscles. As a result of this prevention program, it is estimated that only 1% of the Inuit population of Nunavik is infected with trichinellosis.[27] Toxoplasmosis and congenital toxoplasmosis are also extremely common among the Inuit (http://www.arcticnet-ulaval.ca), with a seroprevalence of approximately 60%.[29] Among the important risk factors are the ingestion of seal and caribou.[29]

Echinococcosis

There are two major forms of the helminth infection known as echinococcosis that affect the Inuit. Cystic echinococcosis, caused by the tapeworm *Echinococcus granulosus*, occurs throughout the North American Arctic, where the natural mammalian hosts of the *E. granulosus* tapeworms are the wolves and sled dogs fed the offal (organ meats) of moose, reindeer, and elk (http://www.arcticnet-ulaval.ca).[30] Humans become infected by a fecal-oral route in which they accidentally ingest the eggs excreted in the feces of sled dogs. Upon ingestion, the eggs liberate larval stages that travel to the lungs and liver, where they produce large fluid-filled cysts. In some patients, the cysts can grow to more than 10 cm in diameter, enabling them to cause mechanical destruction of the affected organs. Alternatively, the cysts can rupture and the leaked fluid can produce severe allergic reactions. The treatment often requires surgical intervention, although anthelmintic drugs such as albendazole appear either to reduce the risks or in some cases to cure the disease entirely. During the first half of the 20th century, when the Inuit led a largely nomadic existence with heavy dependence on sled dogs for travel, cystic echinococcosis was a serious problem. However, as permanent settlements began to develop and as dogs were replaced by snowmobiles and other vehicles, the life cycle of *E. granulosus* was largely interrupted and today the number of cases is small.[30] According to a seroprevalence study (http://www.arcticnet-ulaval.ca) conducted in Nunavik, approximately 12,000 Inuit have been infected with *E. granulosus*.

Alveolar echinococcosis is a second and more severe form. Caused by *Echinococcus multilocularis*, this form of echinococcosis produces cysts which are both highly infiltrative and metastatic and therefore sometimes not treatable by surgical modalities. Alveolar echinococcosis has a high mortality rate. The disease is believed to have been first introduced by arctic foxes and now is endemic in the prairie provinces of Canada as well as in the Dakotas, Montana, and Wyoming.[31] The number of cases that occur annually is not known.

Summary of NTDs in the United States and Canada

Table 9.1 shows a summary of the number of possible cases of NTDs in the United States and Canada. For the most part, these numbers were extrapolated on the basis of very limited data, but I present them here because they point out the potential seriousness of the problem and the urgent need for meaningful surveillance studies.

Table 9.1 Summary of the NTDs of the United States and Canada

Disease	Estimated no. of cases
Giardiasis	424,120–2,120,600
Toxocariasis	323,000–500,000
Chagas' disease	150,000
Strongyloidiasis	68,000
Cysticercosis	2,800–41,400
Cystic echinococcosis	12,000
Congenital toxoplasmosis	400–4,000 per yr
Trichinellosis	1,500
Alveolar echinococcosis	<100
Dengue fever	Not determined
Leptospirosis	Not determined
Trachoma	Not determined

NTDs in Mexico and the Caribbean

High rates of NTDs occur in many regions of rural Mexico, especially in southern Mexico near the borders of Guatemala and Belize. For example, in the southern states of Chiapas and Oaxaca, onchocerciasis is focally endemic, although there are no new cases of blindness because ivermectin has been distributed aggressively in the communities where onchocerciasis is most endemic.[32] In addition, hookworm infection and other soil-transmitted helminth infections are endemic to Chiapas (as well as elsewhere in rural Mexico),[33] trachoma is still focally endemic, and the number of cases of CL has increased because of interruptions in public health control measures forced by guerrilla movements in the region.[34] Chagas' disease still occurs in focal regions of the country, and between 1990 and 2005, 1,532 new acute infections were recorded.[35] However, under a system of active surveillance that used 1.5 million blood samples collected from patients with fever in over 16,000 rural areas, fewer than 10 acute cases were identified annually.[35] Dengue, leptospirosis, and the protozoan infection amebiasis are important infections in Mexico's urban and rural areas.[34]

Although we cannot consider most of the Caribbean a part of the United States, millions of Americans vacation there annually. Today, the Caribbean is considered the most tourism-dependent region in the world, with tourism dollars responsible for an estimated 25% of the region's gross domestic product (http://www.carec.org). However, there is a forgotten side to the Caribbean. High rates of selected NTDs, especially LF, schistosomiasis, hookworm, and dengue, exist in the region. The highest rates of LF occur in Haiti and the Dominican Republic (DR), while the highest rates of schistosomiasis occur in the DR and Guadeloupe.[36] Hookworm infection and other soil-transmitted helminth infections are also endemic to the Caribbean, particularly Haiti and Belize, but overall there are very few present-day data on their prevalence.[37]

Given that tourism generates more than US$30 billion annually in the Caribbean, it is truly shocking that such obvious diseases of poverty, LF and schistosomiasis could be allowed to remain endemic. In the beginning of this book (in chapter 1), I pointed out how hookworm infection, LF, and schistosomiasis represent a historical legacy of the Middle Passage of the Atlantic slave trade from Africa (a link first proposed by Pat Lammie and his colleagues at the CDC and the Pan American Health Organization).[38] It is therefore an especially sad fact that we allow these diseases to remain near where Americans go to play. It is especially remarkable that, if every American who travels to the Caribbean in the next year were to contribute toward NTD control, we would likely have sufficient funds to eliminate LF, schistosomiasis, and possibly other NTDs from the region.

Conclusions

The frequent unavailability of reliable numbers on the prevalence of the NTDs is reflective of their neglected status and of their disproportionate impact on the poorest of the poor. Many of these NTDs could be easily controlled or eliminated and at relatively modest cost. The most immediate need is to support studies in order to better assess the true prevalence of these infections and then to identify simple and cost-effective public health solutions. There are really no excuses for allowing such glaring health disparities to continue in the backyards of some of the world's wealthiest countries.

Summary Points: NTDs in the United States and Canada

- NTDs are common among the minority populations and indigenous peoples of North America, although their true prevalence has not been well studied.
- The major U.S. NTDs include soil-transmitted helminth infections, especially toxocariasis and strongyloidiasis, cysticercosis, Chagas' disease, and toxoplasmosis. Cysticercosis may be the single leading cause of epilepsy in the Southwestern United States, and toxoplasmosis is a major cause of birth defects.
- The Inuit of the Canadian Arctic and Alaska also suffer from several NTDs, including toxoplasmosis, trichinellosis, and echinococcosis.
- Several NTDs, including onchocerciasis, soil-transmitted helminths, trachoma, and CL, occur frequently in rural southern Mexico, especially in Chiapas, and Chagas' disease is still focally endemic.
- Schistosomiasis and LF remain serious, endemic NTDs in the Caribbean.
- The NTDs represent some of North America's greatest health disparities.

chapter 10

The Global Network for Neglected Tropical Disease Control

And it's not just the story about one billion people who are afflicted with disabling, often-times stigmatizing, neglected tropical diseases, such as human hookworm infection and elephantiasis... it's all about the faces of dying children and sick mothers who haunt those who have seen them.

FORMER PRESIDENT BILL CLINTON

Comprehensive, Africa-wide control of malaria and NTDs together would probably cost no more than $3 billion a year, or just two days of Pentagon spending. If each of the billion people in the rich world devoted the equivalent of one $3 coffee a year to the cause, several million children every year would be spared death and debility, and the world would be spared the grave risks when disease and despair run unchecked. A new Global Network for Neglected Tropical Disease Control is helping make this opportunity a reality.

JEFFREY SACHS

My experience has taught me that no movement ever stops or languishes for want of funds. This does not mean that any movement can go on without money, but it does mean that wherever it has good men and true at its helm, it is bound to attract to itself the requisite funds.

MAHATMA GANDHI

The neglected tropical diseases (NTDs) are among the leading disabling conditions of humankind. Because of their disfiguring clinical manifestations and their devastating impact on child development, pregnancy outcome, and productive capacity, the core group of 13 NTDs is responsible for a huge disease burden in the low-income countries of Africa, Asia, and the Americas. It is estimated that the NTDs result in 56.6 million DALYs (disability-adjusted life years, i.e., the number of healthy life years lost from disability or premature

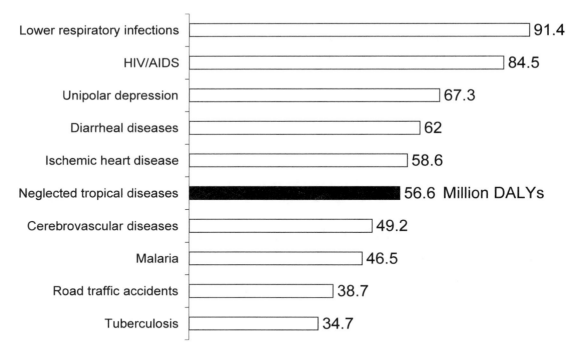

Figure 10.1 The 10 leading causes of DALYs (modified from Hotez et al., 2007b).

death) lost annually. By comparison, this global disease burden exceeds that of malaria and tuberculosis and is almost as great as the number of DALYs lost from HIV/AIDS (Fig. 10.1).[1]

More than 90% of the NTD global disease burden results from the seven most common conditions—ascariasis, trichuriasis, hookworm infection, schistosomiasis, lymphatic filariasis (LF), trachoma, and onchocerciasis. These seven NTDs, which together result in 52.1 million DALYs lost annually, are the most common infections of poor people in developing countries, befalling roughly 40% of the 2.7 billion people who live on less than US$2 per day.[1] Table 10.1 ranks these seven by DALYs and reveals that hookworm and the other soil-transmitted helminth infections top the list, followed by LF, schistosomiasis, trachoma, and onchocerciasis.[1] In the coming years, it is expected that these DALY estimates will be revised through a new initiative sponsored by the Institute of Health Metrics and Evaluation (http://www.healthmetrics-andevaluation.org) under the direction of Chris Murray at the University of Washington in Seattle. Because many of the earlier DALY estimates have not fully considered the chronic features of the NTDs,[2] it is quite possible that our current estimates of disease burden will increase even further.

In addition to their disease burden, through their impact on child cognition, memory, school performance, and school attendance, as well as on worker productivity, the NTDs place an enormous added economic burden on the low-income countries. Although we are still in the nascent stages of

Table 10.1 Ranking of the seven most prevalent NTDs by DALYs[a]

Rank	Disease	Global disease burden: no. of DALYs	Global prevalence
1	Hookworm infection	22.1 million	576 million
2	Ascariasis	10.5 million	807 million
3	Trichuriasis	6.4 million	604 million
4	LF	5.8 million	120 million
5	Schistosomiasis	4.5 million	207 million
6	Trachoma	2.3 million	84 million
7	Onchocerciasis	0.5 million	37 million
	Total	52.1 million	>1 billion

[a]Table modified from Hotez et al., 2006d.

quantifying this economic impact, the information to date suggests that the NTDs represent some of the most important poverty-promoting conditions in developing regions.[3]

An important theme throughout this book has been the concept of mass drug administration (MDA) or preventive chemotherapy. We have seen how the simultaneous administration of NTD drugs to large populations over a defined period can produce dramatic health gains, as well as important educational and economic benefits.[1,3] Proof that this concept would work on large populations was pioneered by the Chinese beginning shortly after the Cultural Revolution, when a part of the nation's salt supply was medicated with diethylcarbamazine (DEC).[1,3] As a result, by the early 1990s, LF was largely eliminated as a public health problem in the People's Republic of China.[1,3] Similarly, MDA with DEC was responsible for the elimination of LF from Egypt and from many of the islands of the South Pacific.[1,3] MDA has also been effective against other NTDs.[1,3] MDA with praziquantel has helped to control schistosomiasis in Egypt, MDA with ivermectin has controlled onchocerciasis in West Africa, and MDA, as part of the SAFE strategy (described in chapter 5), has eliminated trachoma as a public health problem in Morocco.[1,3] Therefore, almost anyone would agree that preventive chemotherapy has significantly cut the global burden of the seven most prevalent NTDs and has resulted in some of the most extraordinary public health victories in the developing world over the last 3 decades.

In recognition of these public health gains, the World Health Assembly has adopted a number of ambitious resolutions over the years to promote the use of MDA for NTDs. Composed of the ministers of health from all 192 member states, the World Health Assembly appoints the director-general of the WHO and is the WHO's major decision-making and health policy-setting body. Of relevance to the seven most prevalent NTDs, the World Health Assembly has adopted four major resolutions involving MDA.[4] They include the elimination of both LF and trachoma as a public health problem by 2020, the establishment of community-based sustainable yearly treatments for onchocerciasis in areas with moderate or high intensity by 2010, and the regular and periodic treatment of at least 75% of school-age children at risk for soil-transmitted helminth infections and schistosomiasis by 2010. Additional World Health Assembly targets are in place for multiple-drug treatments for leprosy and for public health intervention efforts against guinea worm, Chagas' disease, and human African trypanosomiasis.

In order to address these World Health Assembly targets, several very important international public-private partnerships with commitments to NTDs have been established. Table 10.2 gives a summary of the major MDA programs for the seven most prevalent NTDs.[4] Working with the WHO, these major partnerships are currently helping to enable access to essential NTD medicines for the poorest people in low-income countries. The major organizations include:

- *Partners for Parasite Control* (PPC) (http://www.who.int/wormcontrol). The PPC promotes the widespread use of benzimidazole anthelmintics (mebendazole and albendazole) together with praziquantel in order to treat high-risk groups, especially school-age children, for soil-transmitted helminth infections and schistosomiasis. It comprises agencies of the UN, WHO member states, research institutes (including the Sabin Vaccine Institute [http://www.sabin.org]), and nongovernmental organizations (NGOs), with the WHO acting as the secretariat and lead technical agency.
- *Schistosomiasis Control Initiative* (SCI) (http://www.schisto.org). SCI also promotes the sustainable control of schistosomiasis and of some soil-transmitted helminth infections in sub-Saharan Africa by working with health ministries and national control programs to deliver praziquantel and benzimidazole anthelmintics to high-risk groups, especially school-age children. Under the direction of Alan Fenwick, SCI is based at Imperial College, London.
- *Global Alliance to Eliminate Filariasis* (GAELF) (http://www.filariasis.org). GAELF coordinates the activities of partners working to deliver either DEC or ivermectin, together with albendazole, with a focus on political, financial, and technical support. The GAELF Secretariat is currently based at the Liverpool School of Tropical Medicine under the direction of David Molyneux.
- *International Trachoma Initiative* (ITI) (http://www.trachoma.org). ITI is dedicated to the elimination of blinding trachoma through implementation of the SAFE strategy, which includes MDA with azithromycin (Zithromax). ITI was founded by Pfizer and the Edna McConnell Clark Foundation in 1998. The organization is based in New York City and is currently under the direction of interim President Ibrahim Jabr.
- *Helen Keller International* (HKI) (http://www.hki.org). HKI was founded in 1915 and is one of the oldest nonprofit organizations dedicated to fighting and treating preventable malnutrition-caused blindness. Headquartered in New York City, HKI maintains large-scale programs to combat trachoma, onchocerciasis, and other causes of blindness. HKI is under the direction of Kathy Spahn.

Table 10.2 Summary of MDA programs for the most prevalent NTDs[a]

Disease	Major initiatives	Size of at-risk population	Drug(s) used	Frequency	Major target populations
Soil-transmitted helminth infections (ascariasis, trichuriasis, and hookworm infection)	Partnership for Parasite Control (www.who.int/wormcontrol), Schistosomiasis Control Initiative (www.schisto.org), Sabin Vaccine Institute (www.sabin.org), Mebendazole Donation Program (Johnson & Johnson) (www.taskforce.org/mebendazole)	>3 billion people in most of Africa, Southeast Asia, India and South Asia, and tropical Americas	Mebendazole or albendazole	Once or twice/yr depending on prevalence or level of transmission	School-age children and some preschool children and women of reproductive age
Schistosomiasis	Schistosomiasis Control Initiative (www.schisto.org), Partnership for Parasite Control (www.who.int/wormcontrol)	779 million people in 76 countries in Africa, the Middle East, tropical Americas, China, East Asia, and the Pacific	Praziquantel	Once/yr or every 2 yr, or twice during primary school depending on prevalence or level of transmission	School-age children
LF	Global Alliance to Eliminate LF (www.filariasis.org), Albendazole Donation Program (GlaxoSmithKline)	1.3 billion people in 83 countries in Africa, Asia, tropical Americas, and western Pacific	DEC or ivermectin	Once/yr	Entire at-risk population
Onchocerciasis	African Programme for Onchocerciasis Control (www.apoc.bf), Helen Keller International (www.hki.org), Carter Center (www.cartercenter.org), Onchocerciasis Elimination Program for the Americas (ww.who.int/blindness), Mectizan Donation Program (Merck) (www.mectizan.org)	90 million people in Africa, Yemen, and the tropical Americas	Ivermectin	Once/yr	Entire at-risk population
Trachoma	International Trachoma Initiative (www.trachoma.org), Helen Keller International (www.hki.org), Carter Center (www.cartercenter.org)	590 million people in 55 countries in Africa and Asia but also in pockets of the Americas and Australia	Azithromycin	Once/yr	Entire at-risk population ≥ 6 mos. of age

[a]See note 4.

- *African Programme for Onchocerciasis Control* (APOC) (http://www.apoc.
  bf). APOC was founded to eliminate onchocerciasis as a public health
  problem throughout the entire continent. The cornerstone of the organization is CDTI (community drug treatments with ivermectin) working
  through a network of hundreds of thousands of distributors. APOC has a
  broad spectrum of partners, including many nongovernmental development organizations. Its executing agency is the WHO, and its fiscal agency
  is the World Bank. APOC is based in Ouagadougou, Burkina Faso, under
  the direction of Uche Amazigo.
- *Task Force for Child Survival and Development* (Task Force) (http://www.
  taskforce.org). The Task Force houses many of the drug donation programs which work with the partnerships outlined above. They include
  the Mectizan Donation Program (http://www.mectizan.org), linked with
  Merck, and the donation programs for mebendazole (Johnson & Johnson)
  and albendazole (GlaxoSmithKline). The Task Force is based in Atlanta,
  GA, and is under the direction of Mark Rosenberg.
- *Carter Center* (http://www.cartercenter.org). Founded in 1982 by former
  U.S. President Jimmy Carter and former First Lady Rosalynn Carter, in
  partnership with Emory University, the Atlanta-based center works to
  relieve human suffering in more than 70 countries. The Carter Center
  operates major programs in the control of multiple NTDs, including
  guinea worm infestation, onchocerciasis, and trachoma. Its success in
  guinea worm eradication was discussed earlier (in chapter 4).

Through these partnerships, MDA has been scaled to an extraordinary
level, now reaching tens of millions of people who are either infected with
NTDs or at high risk for acquiring NTDs. However, even this level of activity is
probably not sufficient in order to reach the highly ambitious targets for control and elimination set by the World Health Assembly. Over the last 30 years,
it has been estimated that less than one-half of the eligible populations have
received preventive chemotherapy treatments for the soil-transmitted helminth
infections, schistosomiasis, LF, and trachoma. Therefore, at our current rate of
MDA, it could be another century or longer before the world's poorest people
gain full access to the essential medicines for the NTDs.

The hurdles to increasing the level of MDA by the WHO and the major NTD
partnerships are formidable. As pointed out in the beginning of this book, the
global health community, especially the Group of Eight (G8) nations, has not
supported NTD control activities at nearly the same level as it has HIV/AIDS,
malaria, and tuberculosis, relief through the Global Fund, President's Emergency Plan for AIDS Relief (PEPFAR), President's Malaria Initiative (PMI), and
other initiatives. To date, the G8 support of NTD control can be measured
in millions of dollars rather than the billions devoted to control of the big
three diseases.

However, lack of political will has not been the only hurdle to global NTD
control. Given that the NTDs occur primarily in the rural (and often remote)
areas of the developing world, there is a need to make MDA more accessible to

these populations and possibly make it a more efficient enterprise. As we saw earlier (in chapter 5), probably more than any other organization, APOC has been effective at reaching vulnerable populations. By working through a system of community-based drug distributors, APOC is administering ivermectin to some of the most remote and vulnerable rural populations affected by river blindness.

Since APOC is already doing the "hard part," namely, obtaining access to Africa's hardest-to-reach populations, is there a rationale for APOC and similar organizations to administer not only ivermectin but other NTD drugs as well? Color Plate 1 is a map of the world illustrating where the seven most prevalent NTDs occur. The map illustrates an aggregated distribution of these seven conditions. Thus, whereas none of the most common NTDs are public health problems in North America, Europe, and Central Asia, there are multiple NTDs occurring in the tropical developing world, particularly in sub-Saharan Africa, Southeast Asia, and tropical regions of the Americas. In fact, in many countries of these developing regions, it is common to find five, six, or seven of the most highly prevalent NTDs occurring in the same geographic region. In other words, the seven most common NTDs are coendemic in these regions.

To understand better the implications of coendemic NTDs, let us take as an example the nation of Cote d'Ivoire (also known as the Ivory Coast) on the western coast of Africa. Roughly the size of New Mexico, Cote d'Ivoire is a low-income country with a per capita annual income of approximately US$1,500.[5] In addition to high levels of rural poverty and a high rate of infant and under-age-five child mortality, Cote d'Ivoire is facing ongoing civil conflict between the government in the south and the rebels in the north.[5] In 2002, Giovanna Raso, Juerg Utzinger, and their colleagues at the Swiss Tropical Institute, together with scientists from Cote d'Ivoire's Universite de Cocody in Abidjan, conducted a study among 75 randomly selected households in a single rural village where they obtained complete parasitological data on almost all the study participants. They found that three-quarters of the population harbored three or more parasites simultaneously, including hookworms, schistosomes, amebae, and malaria parasites.[6] Practically speaking, this finding means that in rural Cote d'Ivoire, as in many of the areas illustrated in red and orange in Color Plate 1, people living in rural poverty are polyparasitized; i.e., they suffer from multiple NTDs at any given time. In a follow-up study among schoolchildren in Cote d'Ivoire, coinfections with hookworm and schistosomes were found to be particularly common, a finding subsequently confirmed in Brazil.[6] Indeed, the Brazilian studies suggest that infection with hookworm may predispose to schistosomiasis, so that there are synergistic effects as well as additive ones. Thus, investigations in many developing countries have shown that polyparasitism is common, not only because schoolchildren frequently have all three major soil-transmitted helminth infections (the unholy trinity of ascariasis, trichuriasis, and hookworm infection) but also because they have additional coinfections with schistosomiasis, LF, onchocerciasis, and even trachoma.

It is important to understand the full extent of NTD coinfections across sub-Saharan Africa and elsewhere. Accordingly, efforts by a few investigators are under way to employ satellite mapping and geographic information systems in order to overlay the prevalence of specific NTDs with maps of climate and vegetation as a means of predicting the global extent of coinfection and geographic overlap.[7] By folding in behavioral, demographic, and socioeconomic factors, it should become possible to develop complete risk maps for identifying large-scale patterns of potential overlap.[7] However, the evidence emerging to date already indicates that in the poorest rural areas of the developing world, individuals are more frequently than not simultaneously infected with multiple NTDs, typically one or more of the seven most common NTDs.

The facts that the seven NTDs cluster in people and that polyparasitism is common mean that it may be possible to bundle some of the NTD drugs together in a highly cost-effective MDA package. Beginning in 2003, those of us concerned about the plight of polyparasitized populations began to reassess the disease burden associated with the NTDs and opportunities for control. Through a series of meetings held in Europe and the United States, a group of NTD experts who headed partnerships involved in the control of specific NTDs, initially including David Molyneux (GAELF), Alan Fenwick (SCI), and myself, as well as Lorenzo Savioli (director, Department of NTDs, WHO), Vinand Nantulya (Global Fund to Fight AIDS, Tuberculosis, and Malaria), Jacob Kumaresan and Ibrahim Jabr (ITI), Eric Ottesen (Task Force), Frank Richards (Carter Center), Juerg Utzinger (Swiss Tropical Institute), and Jeffrey and Sonia Ehrlich Sachs (Earth Institute at Columbia University), discussed the situation. We identified the following important elements of polyparasitism and opportunities for integrated control.

1. The aggregate NTD health and economic burden is enormous, and the need for a global effort on these diseases is as urgent as the need for major HIV/AIDS and malaria initiatives such as the Global Fund and PEPFAR, to name a few.[8]

2. Because of the high degree of geographic overlap and coendemicity of the NTDs and the high prevalence of polyparasitism, the seven most prevalent NTDs—the three soil-transmitted helminth infections (ascariasis, hookworm infection, and trichuriasis) plus schistosomiasis, LF, trachoma, and onchocerciasis—could be simultaneously targeted with a package of drugs comprising albendazole or mebendazole (targeting primarily the soil-transmitted helminths), praziquantel (for schistosomiasis), ivermectin or DEC (for LF and onchocerciasis), and azithromycin (for trachoma).[9] The package of drugs for integrated NTD control has been named by some the "rapid-impact package" because the drugs can be quickly deployed by community-based drug distributors.[9]

3. Integrated NTD control through the rapid-impact package would be expected to have a number of health impacts, especially for children and women. Among them would be worm burden reductions and reductions in worm-associated anemia from hookworm infection and schistosomiasis; improvements in child growth and development, pregnancy outcome (both in terms of neonatal birth weight and maternal morbidity and

mortality), and worker productivity; and prevention of blindness, chronic disability, and disfigurement.[10] In addition to targeting the seven NTDs, the rapid-impact package would also have an impact on less common helminth infections such as the food-borne trematode infections, strongyloidiasis, taeniasis, some protozoan infections such as giardiasis, and even some ectoparasitic skin infestations such as scabies and pediculosis (lice). The reduction of skin disease from both onchocerciasis and ectoparasites could also prevent secondary complications from cutaneous bacterial infections.[10]

4. The ability of integrated NTD control to reduce anemia is of particular importance. Hookworm infection, trichuriasis, and schistosomiasis all cause anemia, and an important clinical consequence of polyparasitism is enhancement of anemia, particularly in school-age children and pregnant women.[11] Anemia in school-age children results in decreased motor activity, social inattention, and decreased school performance and increases susceptibility to infection.[12] Anemia is also associated with increased maternal morbidity and low neonatal birth weight and accounts for 3.7 and 12.8% of maternal deaths during pregnancy and childbirth in Africa and Asia, respectively.[11, 12] To date, studies have shown that worm burden reduction through deworming improves childhood iron status and reduces anemia in pregnant women, resulting in reductions in the frequency of low birth weight and infant and maternal mortality.[13]

5. In addition to improving health, the integration of NTD control would improve child cognition and educational performance and attendance, as well as promote economic development in the poorest regions on Earth.[14]

6. Through integrated control with the rapid-impact package, health, educational, and economic improvements could be achieved at remarkably low cost. Ivermectin and azithromycin are donated free of charge and for as long as needed by Merck and Pfizer, respectively, while GlaxoSmithKline donates albendazole for LF control, Johnson & Johnson donates some of the mebendazole required for the global control of soil-transmitted helminth control, and Merck KGaA donates some of the praziquantel required for schistosomiasis control. In addition, albendazole, mebendazole, DEC, and praziquantel are available as low-cost generic drugs. MedPharm also donates considerable doses of generic albendazole and praziquantel. Therefore, the costs of purchase and delivery of the drugs comprising the rapid-impact package are extremely modest. Initial estimates suggested that the package could be administered for US$0.50 per person, with other estimates ranging up to US$0.79 per person.[1,15] In either case, as shown in Fig. 10.2, the costs of administering the rapid-impact package are extremely small compared to the annual per-person costs of antiretroviral therapy for HIV/AIDS, direct observed therapy for tuberculosis, or even antimalaria drugs and bed nets.

On a macroeconomic scale, the low cost of integrated NTD control means that the health and education of entire populations can be improved for

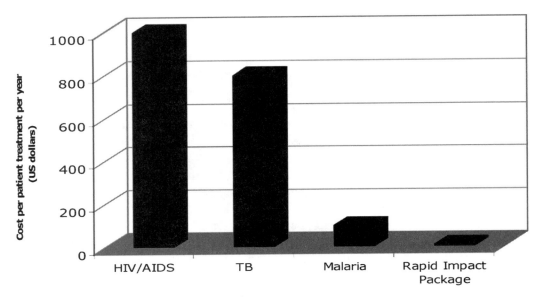

Figure 10.2 Range of treatment costs per person per year for HIV/AIDS, TB, malaria, and the rapid-impact package for integrated NTD control (modified from Molyneux et al., 2005). The rapid-impact package costs as little as US$0.50 per person for packaged intervention. Data derived from previous research (Hotez et al., 2007a).

extremely modest sums of money. For instance, the entire at-risk population of rural sub-Saharan Africa (500 million people) could be treated annually for between $250 million and $400 million.[1,15] Therefore, for US$1 billion to US$2 billion over a period of five years, up to 500 million at-risk people in sub-Saharan Africa could be blanketed with NTD drugs. By the end of the five-year period, it would be expected that substantial reductions in LF and trachoma would be achieved, possibly to the point of elimination in some countries, with substantial morbidity control for soil-transmitted helminth infections (especially ascariasis and trichuriasis for school-age children), schistosomiasis, and onchocerciasis.[15] Compared to an estimated US$3 billion annually for malaria control (which is still very reasonable),[16] the cost of NTD control is ridiculously modest. When one uses a metric known as the dollar per DALY averted, deworming is estimated to cost between US$2 and US$9 per DALY averted,[16] and with an estimated cost savings through integration of up to 47%,[4] this cost would be reduced even further.[1] By comparison, it costs US$150 per DALY averted to treat ischemic stroke with aspirin and US$1,000 or more per DALY averted for higher-technology Western interventions such as the administration of tissue plasminogen activator to prevent restenosis of the coronary arteries.[16] Therefore, according to these estimates, integrated NTD control represents one of the very "best buys" in public health. Harvard's David Canning has further pointed out that integrated NTD control also represents a priority investment in human capital.[17]

Administering the rapid-impact package requires recognition that not all groups should receive the same drugs and at the same time.[18] For instance, the drugs for soil-transmitted infections and schistosomiasis—albendazole, mebendazole, and praziquantel—are intended primarily for school-age (and some preschool) children, while ivermectin and DEC are administered to adult populations and to some children who have reached a specified age or height. Usually DEC is not administered at all for LF control in sub-Saharan Africa, because it is too toxic to patients who are also infected with onchocerciasis, while ivermectin is safe for both LF and onchocerciasis in Africa. Therefore, DEC is primarily reserved for Asian LF and for LF in the Americas. In order to cover many of these contingencies and to tailor the rapid-impact package drugs to situations where some but not all of the NTDs are endemic, the WHO has developed and issued a set of detailed guidelines and algorithms for administering the major NTD drugs to polyparasitized populations.[18]

In order to facilitate integration, many of the NTD partnerships mentioned in the previous chapters, including SCI, GAELF, and ITI, as well as the Earth Institute at Columbia University, the Task Force for Child Survival and Development, and HKI, have joined in an alliance known as the Global Network for Neglected Tropical Disease Control (also known as the Global Network for NTDs or simply the "Global Network").[1] The Secretariat of the Global Network is based at the Sabin Vaccine Institute in Washington, DC (http://www.sabin.org) (Fig. 10.3). The mission of the Global Network and its partners is to help those who suffer from and are at risk for the NTDs through effective collaboration, scaling up of existing disease interventions, and development of a new generation of improved control tools.[19] Our vision is a world free of NTDs in which healthy people can develop fully, learn effectively, raise families, and be productive members of their communities.

Launched at the Clinton Global Initiative in 2006, the Global Network Secretariat focuses its activities primarily on advocacy and resource mobilization in order to achieve the overall goal of increasing access to essential medicines for the estimated 1 billion people affected by NTDs by 2015. Doing so would

Figure 10.3 Logos of the major NTD partnerships comprising the Global Network for NTD Control.

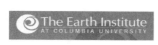
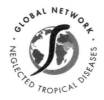
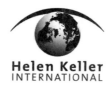
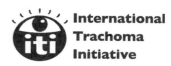
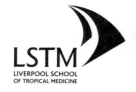
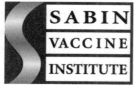
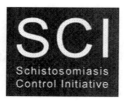
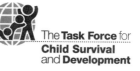

improve childhood development, school attendance and performance, pregnancy outcomes, and worker productivity among the world's poorest populations. Moreover, reduction of the health, educational, and economic burden of the NTDs will directly address the Millennium Development Goals for sustainable poverty reduction in developing countries. In order to promote this advocacy agenda, the Global Network has inaugurated a new website devoted to NTDs, and articles about its activities have appeared in the print and electronic media, including a lead editorial by *New York Times* columnist Nicholas Kristof.[20] Actress Alyssa Milano has also committed her time and energy (and has provided a financial commitment) to the Global Network by agreeing to serve as its inaugural global goodwill ambassador. In time, the Global Network will, together with the WHO, form a full and comprehensive partnership for the control and elimination of the major NTDs.

National programs of integrated control have begun in several African countries, including Burkina Faso, Burundi, Ghana, Mali, Niger, Rwanda, Togo, and Uganda, and in at least two states of Nigeria.[21] Funding for these early NTD integration efforts has come primarily either from the philanthropic investment organization Legatum and Geneva Global, Inc. (administered through the Global Network) or from a congressional appropriation administered through the U.S. Agency for International Development (USAID).[11,19,21] The Carter Center is taking the lead on the two Nigerian states. These nascent efforts at integrated control are expected to produce dramatic gains for the poorest people in these African countries. Monitoring and evaluation of these programs will include both measuring process indicators, including the number of people actually treated, and assessing reductions in NTD prevalence and worm intensity, improvements in anemia and other nutritional parameters, and catch-up growth in children. A high-level forum sponsored by the Global Network in 2006 has revealed a number of exciting benefits from integrated NTD control, including the strengthening of community-based health systems and the African health work force by promoting the activities of community drug distributors from APOC and other control programs. Because schoolteachers can be trained to administer deworming medicines, Africa's schools can also be developed as potent allies for building health systems there.[21] As NTD integration progresses, an important component of monitoring and evaluation will be a careful appraisal of its cost-effectiveness and efforts to determine how NTD control strengthens health systems.[21] Efforts to answer many of these operational questions are being funded by a new grant from the Bill and Melinda Gates Foundation.

The early days of integrated NTD control have also revealed important challenges and hurdles.[21] They include important operational issues, including patient compliance, pharmacological vigilance in using the NTD drugs in combination, and the specter of possible emerging drug resistance. The last is of particular concern, given the likelihood that use of the NTD drugs will become widespread in Africa and elsewhere. This possibility is discussed in more detail later (in chapter 11). We are also facing the enormous hurdle of effecting integrated NTD control in Africa's fragile conflict-ridden and postconflict nation-states. Because of long interruptions in public health control measures caused by the collapse of their health care infrastructures, countries such as Angola, the Central African Republic, Chad, Cote d'Ivoire, the Democratic Republic of the Congo, and Sudan have some of the world's highest NTD prevalence and intensity rates. This issue will be addressed in chapter 12.

Ultimately, as lessons are learned and if the major operational research questions are addressed, integrated control should, in time, become more efficient and streamlined. Assisting in this effort is the exciting possibility of expanding geographic information and remote sensing (GIS/RS) efforts in order to map large areas of sub-Saharan Africa for NTDs.[7,22] Still another exciting opportunity is the prospect of linking NTD control to the control of malaria and other diseases. For example, while working with community ivermectin drug distributors on LF and onchocerciasis control projects in central Nigeria, Frank Richards of the Carter Center and his colleagues from the CDC observed that in areas where MDA was practiced, the ownership and use of antimalarial bed nets dramatically increased, as much as ninefold.[23] Since insecticide-treated nets are considered a major tool in the fight against malaria, it is worth exploring whether there might be other entry points for integrated NTD control to embrace malaria control as a part of its mission or vice versa. Indeed, there is a high degree of geographic overlap and coendemicity of malaria with the major NTDs. For example, Color Plate 16 offers a map of Africa demonstrating the geographic overlap between malaria and hookworm infection.[24] Studies by Simon Brooker and his colleagues at the London School of Tropical Medicine and Hygiene indicate that of the 179 million school-age children living in Africa, approximately 50 million are infected with hookworm and that 90% of these children are at risk for coincident infection with malaria.[24]

The observation of NTD-malaria coendemicity has important implications. Malaria is a leading cause of morbidity and mortality sub-Saharan Africa, and a significant component of malaria's disease burden results from the severe anemia that it causes in both children and pregnant women. If we now superimpose on these two vulnerable malaria-infected populations the blood loss and iron deficiency anemia of hookworm infection, and possibly as well the anemia-causing elements of schistosomiasis, the result is a "perfect storm" of anemia in areas of rural poverty in sub-Saharan Africa.[1] In Kenya, Brooker and his colleagues were able to show that in both preschool children and school-age children, coinfection with malaria and heavy hookworm was associated with significantly worse malaria than were single infections with either malaria or hookworm.[25] Moreover, it is believed that most of the estimated 7.5 million pregnant women in Africa with hookworm are exposed to malaria sometime during their pregnancy, so that coinfection would also exacerbate anemia in this vulnerable population.[26] The term "agriculture-related anemias" has been used to describe the high prevalence of anemia in rural areas of developing countries resulting from the cumulative morbidities of NTDs and malaria and nutritional deficiencies, as well as some common genetic causes of anemia such as sickle-cell diseases and thalassemias.[1,27]

The public health impact of the additive anemia resulting from overlapping NTDs both with and without malaria was described earlier.[1] Briefly, in young children, severe anemia is a leading cause of death, while in older children anemia results in impaired physical growth and cognition and is an important reason why hookworm is such a major global pathogen. Similarly, in pregnant women, anemia is a major contributory factor in low birth weight and even in the death of the mother. Moreover, the morbidities resulting from malaria and helminth coinfections may be synergistic as well as additive. Pierre Druilhe and his colleagues at the Institut Pasteur in Paris have accumulated evidence indicating that selected NTDs, especially schistosomiasis and hookworm infection, may, by modulating the immune system, increase the likelihood of infection with malaria or worsen the number or severity of clinical malaria attacks.[28]

Therefore, an anticipated benefit of linking malaria control and NTD control in Africa would be the major health gains that could result from further reductions in anemia, greater than what would result from NTD control alone, as well as the possible provision of a back-door mechanism to help achieve malaria control. Investigators associated with the Global Network and others have identified a number of possible entry points for linking malaria control with NTD control.[29] They include both mosquito vector control measures and simultaneous administration of antimalaria and NTD drugs. With regard to the former in rural sub-Saharan Africa, LF is transmitted by the same *Anopheles* species that transmits malaria parasites, so insecticide-treated bed nets used to control malaria can also be used to prevent LF.[21,29] Moreover, anthelmintic drugs used during pregnancy to reduce anemia from hookworm could be used alongside a recommended regimen of antimalaria drugs known as intermittent preventive therapy (IPT) of pregnancy, in which administration of a curative regimen of sulfadoxine-pyrimethamine (SP) after 20 weeks of pregnancy is followed by a second dose at least 1 month later.[25] IPT is now a WHO-recommended strategy for the prevention of malaria-related maternal anemia and low birth weight; it is also being investigated as an approach for malaria control in children.[29]

Linking malaria control with NTD control is expected to provide for more efficient use of the limited funds available for vulnerable populations, while at the same time maximizing involvement of the community. Therefore, I feel that the major malaria experts and policymakers need to recognize the potential for enhanced access through NTD control measures, particularly because it could be achieved at minimal cost. Jeffrey Sachs and I have estimated that the cost of NTD control would add only 10% to estimated malaria control costs.[30] This is a very modest investment, given the return in terms of anemia reduction and enhanced bed net use and other operational synergies.

In addition to its contribution to malaria prevention, there are reasons to believe that NTD control could have an impact on the global HIV/AIDS epidemic.[31] Zvi Bentwich and his colleagues in Israel have shown that parasitic worms affect the host immune system in such a manner that they cause people already infected with HIV/AIDS to have larger amounts of virus in their system.[31] These studies have been confirmed in baboons coinfected with schistosomes and HIV.[31] Further, there is now evidence that in women urinary schistosomiasis also affects the genital tract. Studies conducted by a Norwegian group of scientists have shown that such schistosome-infected women have a threefold increase in risk of contracting the AIDS virus, while additional investigations have shown that worms also increase the likelihood of virus passing from mother to baby.[31] Therefore, it may turn out that NTD control may be a key not only for malaria control but for HIV/AIDS control as well.

The important coendemic and synergistic effects of the NTDs on malaria and HIV/AIDS in Africa, and possibly elsewhere, suggest that a key opportunity is being overlooked in the failure to embrace NTD control as part of the global agenda to fight the big three diseases. As I indicated in the beginning of this book, the G8 nations have pumped billions of dollars into large-scale treatment programs for the big three. The largest funding instrument is the Global Fund to Fight AIDS, Tuberculosis, and Malaria. As of 2007, the Global Fund has committed US$7.7 billion in 136 countries to support antiretroviral therapies to treat HIV/AIDS, direct observed therapies for tuberculosis, and antimalaria drugs and bed nets (http://www.theglobalfund.org). With the appointment in 2007 of Harvard-educated French physician Michel Kazatchkine as its new executive director, and with the largest contribution ever by the U.S. government (U.S. financing is now reaching $3 billion), the Global Fund has gained additional momentum. The coendemicity and the operational synergies between AIDS, malaria, and the NTDs argue strongly for including low-cost and cost-effective NTD control measures in the next round of the Global Fund, as well as large-scale bilateral initiatives from the U.S. government such as PEPFAR and PMI. As an alternative scenario, we could establish a stand-alone NTD drug fund in order to ensure that the world's poorest people receive access to these essential medicines. I believe strongly that these topics deserve discussion at the next G8 summit. I am also hopeful that, through the Global Network and other advocacy organizations, the coming years could be remembered for catapulting the NTDs to the attention of global health and poverty advocates everywhere.

Summary Points: the Global Network

- The seven most prevalent NTDs—ascariasis, trichuriasis, hookworm infection, schistosomiasis, LF, trachoma, and onchocerciasis—exhibit a high degree of geographic overlap and coendemicity, especially in sub-Saharan Africa.
- In areas of coendemicity, populations are frequently polyparasitized, creating the opportunity to simultaneously target multiple NTDs with a package of drugs.
- A rapid-impact package of drugs—comprising either albendazole or mebendazole; DEC or ivermectin; praziquantel; and azithromycin—has been designed to target the seven most common NTDs. The drugs are given in different combinations according to WHO preventive chemotherapy guidelines.

Summary Points *(continued)*

- Because many of the drugs are donated, the rapid-impact package is both extremely inexpensive and highly cost-effective and can be administered for approximately US$0.50 per person per year. It represents one of the best buys in public health because of its health, educational, and economic impact.
- The Global Network for NTD Control was established to coordinate the NTD integration activities of the major NTD partnerships.
- Integrated control of the NTDs is under way in at least seven sub-Saharan African countries.
- The NTDs also exhibit coendemicity with malaria and HIV/AIDS. There are both theoretical and practical reasons to link NTD control programs with malaria and HIV/AIDS control programs, including the Global Fund.

Future Trends in Control of Neglected Tropical Diseases and the Antipoverty Vaccines

We've begun to share the promise of modern medicine with those suffering from river blindness, sleeping sickness, and other age-old diseases. A handful of innovative, compassionate people around the world have joined forces to develop new drugs for neglected diseases.

SEN. EDWARD KENNEDY

The main obstacle to responding to the needs of those suffering is insufficient incentive for companies to produce drugs that treat and prevent neglected tropical diseases.

SEN. SAM BROWNBACK

A scientist who is also a human being cannot rest while knowledge which might reduce suffering rests on the shelf.

ALBERT B. SABIN

The seven most prevalent neglected tropical diseases (NTDs) (in order of prevalence, they are ascariasis, trichuriasis, hookworm infection, schistosomiasis, lymphatic filiarisis [LF], trachoma, and onchocerciasis) are the most common infections of the world's poorest people. As a group, they cause disease and disability on a scale that rivals HIV/AIDS or malaria. These conditions also represent a major cause of economic underdevelopment, as they presently block the escape from poverty for the poorest people on our planet. Because integrated NTD control through widespread use of the rapid-impact package of drugs is expected either to reduce the morbidity and disease burdens of the seven most prevalent NTDs or in some cases result in their elimination, it is likely that this approach will become an important ally in the fight for sustainable poverty reduction.

In the previous chapter, I outlined some of the challenges facing large-scale deployment of the rapid-impact package, including the possibility of emerging drug resistance. My concerns about resistance to drugs and other chemical agents stem partly from what we know about the mixed legacy of mass drug administration in the fight against malaria that began shortly after World War II. Widespread use of the insecticide DDT (dichlorodiphenyltrichloroethane) was instrumental in eliminating malaria from much of southern Europe and helped to stimulate economic growth in Greece, Italy, and Spain during the late 1940s and into the 1950s.[1] On the other hand, in some regions of intense malaria endemicity, such as India or sub-Saharan Africa, this same approach has failed.[2] In India throughout the 1950s, mass administration of the antimalarial drug chloroquine, together with intensive spraying of DDT, resulted in the reduction of malaria incidence from an estimated 75 million cases to only 50,000 cases by 1961. As a result of these successes, by the early 1960s there was considerable talk within the global health community and among policymakers about the eventual eradication of malaria in India and, possibly, worldwide. However, the emergence of chloroquine and DDT resistance almost completely reversed these early successes, so that by 1977 there were again tens of millions of malaria cases in India.[2]

This sobering lesson requires us to give serious consideration to the possibility that in areas of high parasite transmission, resistance to some of the drugs being used in the rapid-impact package could also emerge. With plans under way through our Global Network to scale up integrated control interventions for more than 1 billion people living in 56 developing countries where multiple NTDs are coendemic, we need to carefully consider the specter of resistance. Because helminth parasites have much longer replication times than do viruses, bacteria, or even a protozoan organism such as the malaria parasite, we can expect that resistance probably will not emerge as rapidly.[3] However, this observation alone is no excuse for complacency.

Of the six possible different drugs contained in the rapid-impact package—azithromycin, praziquantel, albendazole or mebendazole, and diethylcarbamazine or ivermectin—the agents albendazole and mebendazole particularly stand out as drugs that could induce resistance. Both albendazole and mebendazole belong to the benzimidazole class of compounds. Benzimidazoles similar to albendazole and mebendazole are used widely to deworm ruminant livestock of their soil-transmitted helminths. The gastrointestinal helminth infections of sheep and cattle are both costly veterinary public health and economic problems and are a major reason why it is difficult and sometimes impossible to maintain these animals in an acceptable state of health in many subtropical and tropical countries. For decades, livestock producers in the Southern Hemisphere, especially in South America, South Africa, Australia, and New Zealand, have relied heavily on frequent and periodic treatments with benzimidazole anthelmintics to ensure that their animals harbor low worm burdens throughout the year. Today, however, resistance to benzimidazole is widespread in many parts of the Southern Hemisphere and elsewhere, and in such regions these agents are no longer effective. Resistance to benzimidazole now actually thwarts livestock production in many areas of the world.[4]

Could similar problems emerge among human helminth parasites? For most, if not all, parasitic nematode species, resistance to benzimidazoles results from a point mutation in the parasite genes encoding a protein known as beta-tubulin. Presumably, the benzimidazoles exert their drug effect by binding to beta-tubulin contained in the worm, so that a mutation reduces binding and prevents the drug from acting on the parasite. For the veterinary nematodes, it has been determined that a specific point mutation in the beta-tubulin gene can produce an amino acid change of a phenylalanine to a tyrosine residue in either of two positions in the beta-tubulin gene product, which appears to be sufficient to reduce benzimidazole binding and cause resistance.[5] This benzimidazole resistance-associated mutation was also found in *Wuchereria bancrofti*, the major cause of LF,[5] possibly in association with scaled-up use of albendazole and ivermectin combinations. At the same time, although the resistant phenotype has not yet been conclusively demonstrated for hookworm beta-tubulins, there is evidence demonstrating that mebendazole often is ineffective against hookworms in some parts of the world, especially where the drug has been used frequently.[5] Recently, Nilanthi de Silva of Kelaniya University in Sri Lanka completed an unpublished analysis showing that the cure rates of mebendazole against hookworm can be as low as 9%. Moreover, it has been shown that the efficacy of mebendazole actually worsens with frequent and increasing use.[5] These observations suggest the possibility that resistance has occurred in hookworms as well as in filariae. There is also a suggestion that resistance to ivermectin may have emerged in Ghana in association with widespread use of that drug for onchocerciasis control.[6]

The occurrence of sporadic instances of drug resistance in treatment of human hookworm and filarial worm infections in Africa (and possibly elsewhere) should not deter us from aggressively working to widely deploy rapid-impact packages in developing countries. Drug resistance to helminths does not evolve as rapidly as it does for bacterial and viral pathogens, and in reality, what choice is there? In my opinion, it would be a moral outrage to withhold essential medicines from the world's poorest people because of theoretical concerns about emerging drug resistance. Instead, the best possible approach is to get the existing rapid-impact drugs out to the people who urgently need them, but at the same time recognize the urgency of monitoring for the possible emergence of new pockets of drug resistance. In this regard, a new single-nucleotide polymorphism technique has been developed that could be used to detect benzimidazole resistance among human nematodes.[7]

Concurrently, we need to continue research and development efforts for a new pipeline of anthelmintic drugs. As new drugs are developed, they could be folded into the rapid-impact package when necessary. To date, there are at least three drugs that should be undergoing additional development and testing in the eventual likelihood that they could be folded into the rapid-impact package. One such promising drug out of China is an anthelmintic drug known as tribendimidine. Another is a new class of amino-acetonitrile derivatives from Novartis. While more extensive testing is needed, to date tribendimidine and the amino-acetonitriles appear as though they could one day be used for the mass treatment of soil-transmitted helminth infections.[8] Similarly, the drug moxidectin, developed by Wyeth for veterinary nematodes, may in time become a useful new drug for onchocerciasis, while a new generation of anti-*Wolbachia*-based therapies that target filarial endosymbionts required for effective parasite replication could eventually offer an entirely new approach to the treatment of both onchocerciasis and LF.[8] Additional upstream approaches for developing new anthelmintic drugs also hold promise.[9]

A major obstacle to the development and clinical testing of tribendmi-dine, amino-acetonitriles, moxidectin, new anti-*Wolbachia* compounds, or really for any NTD drug is the total absence of a viable commercial market and therefore the absence of incentive for pharmaceutical companies to embark on anthelmintic drug development projects. Although the major pharmaceutical companies have been willing to donate selected products free of charge in order to combat NTDs in developing countries, it is difficult for a publicly held company responsible to shareholders to take the next step and commit precious resources toward extensive research into and development of new NTD products. As a result, we are faced with a pathetic situation in which out of a total of 1,556 new chemical entities marketed between 1975 and 2004, only 21 drugs were for tropical diseases.[10] Of these, 11 drugs were for malaria or tuberculosis, which have some North American and European markets. This leaves a total of 10 products developed specifically for NTDs over the last 30 years, or roughly 0.6% of the total products developed. The Global Forum for Health Research has coined the term "10/90" to describe the observation that only 10% of global funding for medical research and development is spent on problems that mostly affect the poorest 90% of people in developing countries. In the case of the NTDs, it is more like a 1/99 or a 1/199 gap!

The drug products developed for NTDs since 1975 are listed in Table 11.1. For the most part, they were created by the large, multinational pharmaceutical companies. In at least two cases, the drugs were discovered and developed for a lucrative market for livestock antiparasitic drugs and then later the company supported the development of these drugs as human anthelmintics. This includes the original investment by Merck in ivermectin as a veterinary product and its subsequent, welcomed support of important clinical testing in Africa in order to demonstrate ivermectin's efficacy against onchocerciasis, as well as the discovery and development of albendazole as a veterinary product by the Animal Health division of South Kline & French, before it was subsequently developed by GlaxoSmithKline as a human anthelmintic in 1987. In addition, Bayer AG in Germany developed praziquantel and nifurtimox, Pfizer developed oxamniquine (although this drug has been largely replaced by praziquantel), and now Sanofi-Aventis has taken on the industrial development and distribution of all three major drugs for human African trypanosomiasis—eflornithine, melarsoprol, and pentamidine. Several multinationals have also recently created small neglected-disease divisions, with Novartis taking the step of actually creating an institute for NTDs which emphasizes discovering small-molecule drugs for dengue and tuberculosis.[11]

Table 11.1 New drugs developed between 1975 and 2004 specifically targeting NTDs[a]

Disease	Drug
Ascariasis, trichuriasis, hookworm	Albendazole
Schistosomiasis	Praziquantel
	Oxamniquine
Onchocerciasis, LF	Ivermectin
Leishmaniasis	Liposomal amphotericin B[b]
	Miltefosine
Chagas' disease	Benznidazole
	Nifurtimox
Human African trypanosomiasis	Eflornithine
	Pentamidine isetionate[b]

[a]Modified from Chirac and Torreele, 2006.
[b]These drugs are not new chemical entities but rather a new salt, formulation, or combination.

Given the complete lack of commercial incentive for developing NTD drugs, it is amazing to me that the pharmaceutical world has taken on even this modest degree of research and development. Mary Moran of the London School of Economics and Political Science has undertaken an analysis of the NTD drug pipeline and has identified some interesting factors that could stimulate a multinational company to consider a program of neglected-disease drug and vaccine development.[12] Such incentives are largely based on longer-term business considerations, including corporate social responsibilities and ethical concerns, the strategic consideration of securing better access to developing-country markets and researchers from developing countries, and company reputation.[12] While attending the launch in 2006 of Scientists without Borders, a new nonprofit venture launched by the New York Academy of Sciences (http://www.nyas.org/programs/borders.asp), I was impressed by an evening speech delivered by Jean-Pierre Garnier, the chief executive officer of GlaxoSmith-Kline. He indicated that profit alone was not a sufficient motivation for his tens of thousands of employees to come to work every day. Instead, the employees are partly driven by the knowledge that their company is a leader in helping people in need everywhere.

Despite some track record of developing new drugs for NTDs, it is unreasonable to think that there will be a significant improvement in research and development capacity for new agents if we rely on multinational companies alone. Even with enticements and entitlements for developing NTD products, such as the innovative prospect of advance market commitments proposed by Harvard's Michael Kremer and MIT's Rachel Glennerster or a very timely amendment recently passed by the Senate, the Brownback-Brown Elimination of Neglected Diseases Amendment of the Food and Drug Administration Revitalization Act,[13] it is unlikely that these so-called "pull mechanisms" will by themselves ensure a robust pipeline of new NTD drugs or other health products such as vaccines and diagnostics. It is my prediction that these efforts could become effective in providing important incentives for multinational corporations to take on projects for diseases with both industrialized- and developing-country markets, such as HIV/AIDS, malaria, and tuberculosis, but that they will be less effective at persuading the multinationals to take on de novo projects for diseases that exclusively afflict the world's poorest people.

I believe that, to create a truly robust pipeline of NTD drugs, we also need to look to either smaller biopharmaceutical companies such as AEterna Zentaris GmbH (http://aeternazentaris.com/en/), based in Frankfurt, Germany, which is producing miltefosine, the first oral agent for visceral leishmaniasis, or to a new generation of NTD product development partnerships (PDPs) (also known as public-private partnerships). The PDPs are defined by Mary Moran as "public-health-driven not-for-profit organizations that drive neglected-disease drug development in conjunction with industry groups".[12] Within the last decade, several major PDPs, including some that are based in university-linked research institutes, have been established for research, development, and clinical testing of new drugs for human kinetoplastid infections, e.g., Chagas' disease, human African trypanosomiasis, and leishmaniasis. The major PDPs for new kinetoplastid drugs are listed in Table 11.2.

Table 11.2 PDPs for new drugs to treat human kinetoplastid infections

Organization	Location (headquarters)	President/CEO/director	URL
Drugs for Neglected Diseases Initiative	Geneva, Switzerland	Bernard Pecoul	www.dndi.org
Foundation for Innovative New Diagnostics	Geneva, Switzerland	Giorgio Roscigno	www.finddiagnostics.org
Institute for One World Health	San Francisco, CA	Victoria Hale	www.oneworldhealth.org
Consortium on Human African Trypanosomiasis	Chapel Hill, NC	Richard Tidwell	www.sph.unc.edu
Sandler Center for Basic Research in Parasitic Diseases at UCSF	San Francisco, CA	James McKerrow	www.ucsf.edu/mckerrow
University of Dundee School of Life Sciences Research	Dundee, Scotland	Alan Fairlamb	www.drugdiscovery.dundee.ac.uk
McGill University Department of Microbiology and Immunology	Montreal, Canada	Greg Matlashewski	www.mcgill.ca/microimm
Seattle Biomedical Research Institute	Seattle, WA	Kenneth Stuart	www.sbri.org

These PDPs are either exploiting just-finished genome projects for protozoan parasites,[14] in order to identify potential drug targets, or are embarking on high-throughput screening and other traditional approaches to drug development and clinical testing.[15] Some of these PDPs are supported partly by the Bill and Melinda Gates Foundation. PDPs are presently driving the development and clinical testing of several new antiprotozoan drugs for leishmaniasis and human African trypanosomiasis, including paromomycin, sitamaquine, imiquimod, and pafuramidine maleate, as well as combinations of existing drugs such as nifurtimox-eflornithine and paromomycin-antimonials.[15]

Nascent activities are also in place to develop vaccines to combat the NTDs. I have coined the term "antipoverty vaccines" to emphasize the poverty-promoting features of the NTDs and the impact that such vaccines would have not only on improving global public health, but also on preventing the socioeconomic consequences of these conditions.[16] As shown in Table 11.3, at least five organizations are presently developing NTD vaccines for clinical testing.[16] These include the Institut Pasteur, which is testing a new recombinant vaccine for schistosomiasis, and four PDPs funded completely or partially by the Bill and Melinda Gates Foundation.[16,17] To briefly summarize these projects:

- *Schistosomiasis vaccine.* A team at the Institut Pasteur in Lille, France, has developed a vaccine for urinary schistosomiasis comprised of *Sh*28GST, a recombinant vaccine comprised of a glutathione *S*-transferase derived from *Schistosoma haematobium.* The vaccine is undergoing clinical trials in Niger and Senegal. Other vaccines are under development at the Queensland Institute of Medical Research and in collaboration with the Sabin Vaccine Institute.
- *Leishmaniasis vaccine.* The nonprofit Infectious Disease Research Institute (IDRI), based in Seattle, WA, has developed a new recombinant protein vaccine for leishmaniasis which is undergoing phase 1 clinical testing in

Table 11.3 PDPs for antipoverty vaccines to combat NTDs

Organization	Location	President/Head/ Director	Disease target(s)	Website
Sabin Vaccine Institute	Washington, DC	Peter Hotez	Hookworm, schistosomiasis	www.sabin.org
Infectious Disease Research Institute	Seattle, WA	Steve Reed	Leishmaniasis, leprosy	www.idri.org
Institut Pasteur	Lille, France	Andre and Monique Capron	Schistosomiasis	www.pasteur-lille.fr
Pediatric Dengue Vaccine Initiative	Seoul, Korea	Harold Margolis	Dengue	www.pdvi.org
Fraunhofer USA Center for Molecular Biotechnology	Newark, DE	Rainer Fischer	Nagana (bovine trypanosomiasis)	www.fraunhofer-cmb .org

Brazil and Peru. The belief in the feasibility of a leishmaniasis vaccine is based partly on an ancient practice of "leishmanization" that predates vaccination in some parts of the Middle East and Central Asia, where it was observed that inoculation in the buttocks with live *Leishmania* parasites would prevent disfiguring cutaneous lesions from appearing on the face. IDRI is working to replace live *Leishmania* parasites with a recombinant polyprotein containing three candidate antigen components; the polyprotein is formulated with monophosphoryl lipid A to help the vaccine stimulate protective immunity.[16,17] The leishmaniasis vaccine is being used in combination with anti-*Leishmania* drugs in order to develop safer and shorter treatment regimens.

- *Human hookworm vaccine.* The Human Hookworm Vaccine Initiative (HHVI) is a PDP of the nonprofit Sabin Vaccine Institute in Washington, DC. HHVI-Sabin (also known as HHVI-Sabin Vaccine Institute) works with research, development, manufacturing, and clinical testing units at the George Washington University, the Queensland Institute of Medical Research, and the London School of Hygiene and Tropical Medicine, together with Brazil's FIOCRUZ (Oswaldo Cruz Foundation) and Instituto Butantan, to develop several recombinant vaccine candidates for hookworm infection. These potential vaccines are presently undergoing phase 1 clinical testing in a region of Minas Gerais State, Brazil, where hookworm infection is endemic. The rationale for developing a hookworm vaccine is based on the concerns about drug failures with mebendazole and emerging resistance to benzimidazole described above, together with the proof of concept that it is possible to vaccinate animals with radiation-attenuated infective hookworm larvae.[16,17] HHVI is reproducing the protective immunity that resulted from earlier-generation vaccines by replacing live attenuated organisms with genetically engineered recombinant proteins produced either in bacteria or in yeast. The final human hookworm vaccine will comprise a recombinant protein expressing an infective larval antigen, a recombinant protein expressing an adult hookworm antigen, and a platform adjuvant immunostimulant. It is possible that the human hookworm vaccine will be administered following deworming (sometimes referred to as "vaccine-linked chemotherapy") in order to reduce the likelihood of hookworm reinfection.[18] HHVI is also exploring the possibility of combining hookworm and schistosomiasis vaccines.
- *Dengue vaccine.* The Pediatric Dengue Vaccine Initiative, based at the International Vaccine Institute in Seoul, Korea, is developing an attenuated tetravalent (four dengue virus serotypes) vaccine.[17] The vaccine has successfully entered phase 1 and 2 clinical trials in the United States and Southeast Asia. One of the hurdles to dengue vaccine clinical development is the theoretical concern that if antibody to all four serotypes does not develop following immunization, the recipient could be placed at increased risk of dengue hemorrhagic fever.
- *Nagana (bovine trypanosomiasis) vaccine.* The Fraunhofer USA Center for Molecular Biotechnology uses an innovative plant-based platform

technology to develop a recombinant trypanosome tubulin vaccine against bovine trypanosomiasis.

- *Other vaccines.* Although not organized into PDPs, there are several earlier-stage efforts in place to develop vaccines against other NTDs.[16] For bacterial vaccines, these activities include the early-stage development of a vaccine against leptospirosis based at FIOCRUZ; a joint leprosy vaccine effort between IDRI and the American Leprosy Mission; several early-stage Buruli vaccine efforts, including one based at the Institut Pasteur in Brussels; and *Chlamydia* vaccine efforts based at GlaxoSmithKline in collaboration with other organizations, as well as one based at the University of California–Irvine. The *Chlamydia* vaccines target both genital *Chlamydia* and trachoma. Antiprotozoan vaccine efforts against amebiasis and Chagas' disease have been initiated. Improvements to existing rabies vaccines are in progress. In collaboration with the New York Blood Center and other entities, HHVI-Sabin is exploring the development of a vaccine to combat onchocerciasis, while in collaboration with the Queensland Institute of Medical Research (Australia), a schistosomiasis vaccine development project is being planned. Finally, Novartis has committed some resources to developing vaccines for neglected diseases through a new global health institute that was launched in Siena, Italy, in 2008.

One of the great challenges that face all PDPs is the requirement of following industry practices and engaging federal regulatory bodies such as the U.S. Food and Drug Administration while conducting these activities in the nonprofit sector.[19] For instance, to develop the human hookworm vaccine, HHVI-Sabin conducts process development consisting of scale-up fermentation and protein purification; formulation and potency testing; an extensive documentation system that includes standard operating procedures, protocols, and batch production records; and rigorous quality control and quality assurance standards. HHVI also uses these elements to detail steps for the transfer of these technologies to a manufacturer that can reproduce the process under so-called current Good Manufacturing Practices (cGMP).[19] Following a careful analysis of the manufactured product through lot release and stability testing, it is necessary to submit specific information about the product to an appropriate and internationally recognized regulatory agency (such as the Food and Drug Administration) in order to obtain permission for beginning "first in humans" testing of a new product. Such a phase 1 study is conducted under current Good Clinical Practices (cGCP).

In the preface to this book, I mentioned that, after some 25 years of heading a hookworm research team that in the last few years has successfully developed hookworm antigens as recombinant products for clinical trials, I have begun to realize that this activity is, in some respects, just a beginning exercise. I make this statement because of a terrible record of getting high-technology products such as recombinant vaccines into the hands of vaccinators in developing countries. For instance, it required some 30 years after its discovery for the hepatitis B vaccine to be used widely in some developing countries. Today, it is still not used in many low-income countries in Africa and elsewhere.[20] During the past 30 years, countless thousands of people, particularly in East Asia, have unnecessarily suffered the consequences of chronic hepatitis B infection, including liver failure and liver cancer. One of the major reasons for this lag was cost. When it was first produced, hepatitis B vaccine, a recombinant vaccine produced in genetically engineered yeast, was expensive (over US$100). The high price of the original recombinant hepatitis B vaccine allowed the manufacturer to recover its research, development, and manufacturing costs.[20] Only now are public sector manufacturers in developing countries, such as the Instituto Butantan (Sao Paulo, Brazil), producing hepatitis B vaccine for less than US$1. I worry that decades also will pass before the new human papillomavirus vaccine to prevent cervical cancer comes down from approximately US$360 for the full series of shots to a price suitable for poor women in the developing world. If 30 years is again required, we are facing the prospect of hundreds of thousands of poor women (who do not have access to routine Pap smear screening) needlessly dying of cervical cancer.

Therefore, a principal rationale for my starting HHVI-Sabin was to produce a vaccine that would be low-cost from the very beginning. For it to be cost-effective, we estimate that the human hookworm vaccine (likely a "bivalent product," meaning that it will contain at least two recombinant antigens, each encoding a larval- and adult-stage antigen) will need to be produced for less than US$1. This requirement compels us to build in low-cost manufacturing processes from the very beginning, including the use of inexpensive expression hosts, such as bacteria or yeast, rather than the more expensive mammalian or insect cell lines. It also requires us to produce these products in high volume and to use low-cost column resins to purify the recombinant antigens.

Each of these activities represents a key component of what is referred to now as global access.[21] The NTD PDPs, whether they focus on drug, vaccine, or diagnostic test development, must consider from day one how their products might be used for large numbers of impoverished people. HHVI-Sabin Vaccine Institute has developed a detailed Global Access Roadmap in order to plan how its vaccines will be developed and tested in resource-poor settings. For HHVI-Sabin, an important component of global access is partnering with vaccine manufacturers in middle-income countries where hookworm is endemic. Several of these countries, such as Brazil, China, Cuba, India, Indonesia, Iran, Senegal, and others, have some degree of sophistication in manufacturing health products, including vaccines. Brazil's Carlos Morel and his colleagues refer to such countries as IDCs (innovative developing countries), with innovation defined by quantitatively measuring peer-reviewed papers, international patents, and biotechnology capacity.[22] To ensure global access, HHVI-Sabin Vaccine Institute is transferring its technology for vaccine development to Brazil's Instituto Butantan for scale-up manufacture for the Americas and then possibly for Lusophone Africa (e.g., Angola, Guinea-Bissau, and Mozambique). Simultaneously, HHVI-Sabin partners with FIOCRUZ, roughly Brazil's equivalent of a combined U.S. National Institutes of Health and CDC, for clinical testing in a region of Minas Gerais State where hookworm is endemic. I believe that partnerships with IDCs and low-income countries represent one of the very best opportunities to promote Southern Hemispheric ownership and to ensure global access to new NTD drugs, vaccines, and diagnostics.

With genomes completed for a large number of NTD pathogens, including the agents that cause Chagas' disease, human African trypanosomiasis, leishmaniasis, leprosy, leptospirosis, LF, schistosomiasis, and trachoma, it should be theoretically possible to mine bioinformatics databases in order to develop a large number of antipoverty vaccines in the coming decade. The financier Mike Milken has helped to popularize the phrase "financial innovation" (http://www.milkeninstitute.org). We have the technology in hand to develop new antipoverty drugs, vaccines, and diagnostics, but it is financial innovation that is most needed in order to promote institutions for conducting scale-up process development, manufacturing, and clinical testing and for securing global access for these new products. At the 59th World Health Assembly, the world's health ministers called for increased access to innovation and intellectual property as an important component of the global health agenda. The G8 nations need to do more to finance research, development, and clinical testing of new health products for NTDs and to support resolutions for addressing the 1/199 gap. Among the initiatives under consideration are the possible establishment of a global NTD drug fund; mechanisms folding NTDs into the Global Fund to Fight AIDS, Tuberculosis, and Malaria; and the International Finance Facility for Neglected Diseases (IFFnd).

At the same time, we need to do a better job of developing health system infrastructures so that these new drugs, vaccines, and diagnostics can be folded into NTD rapid-impact packages once they are developed. The control and elimination of the NTDs as a means for sustainably reducing poverty and meeting Millennium Development Goal targets will depend on how successful we are at scaling up integrated NTD control through providing access to existing essential medicines together with access to innovation, so that new products can be incorporated into a new-generation rapid-impact package combining multidimensional health products including drugs, vaccines, and diagnostics. Ultimately, this comprehensive health package will need to be linked with malaria and HIV/AIDS control measures in a holistic and integrated infectious disease control initiative. A road map for advancing this agenda at the scientific and technical level would not be simple, but it is almost definitely feasible. Our far greater challenges are financial innovation and global political will.

Summary Points: Future Trends and the Antipoverty Vaccines

- Because widespread use of the rapid-impact package of drugs is expected to reduce the morbidity and disease burdens of the seven most prevalent NTDs, it is likely that this approach will become an important ally in the fight for sustainable poverty reduction.
- Of the six different drugs contained in the rapid-impact package, albendazole, mebendazole, and ivermectin are potentially vulnerable to drug resistance.
- As alternative agents for the rapid-impact package, tribendimidine, moxidectin, and the anti-*Wolbachia* therapies are under development.
- A major obstacle to the development and clinical testing of NTD drugs is the total absence of commercial incentive. Of a total of 1,556 new chemical entities marketed between 1975 and 2004, only 10 drugs were for NTDs, most of which were developed by multinationals.
- To create a truly robust pipeline of NTD drugs, we need to look to either small biopharmaceuticals or a new generation of NTD PDPs. Many of the NTD PDPs are funded in part by the Bill and Melinda Gates Foundation.
- Within the last decade, several important NTD PDPs have been established for research, development, and clinical testing of new drugs for Chagas' disease, human African trypanosomiasis, and leishmaniasis.
- At least five PDPs have also successfully developed NTD vaccines, also known as antipoverty vaccines, for clinical testing. These include the Institut Pasteur, which is testing a new recombinant vaccine for schistosomiasis; IDRI, which is testing a recombinant vaccine for leishmaniasis; the Pediatric Dengue Vaccine Initiative; the Fraunhofer USA Center for Molecular Biotechnology, which is developing a vaccine for cattle trypanosomiasis; and HHVI-Sabin, which is developing hookworm and schistosomiasis vaccines. These PDPs are producing low-cost vaccines from the outset.
- An important component of global access for health products in developing countries is partnering with manufacturers in middle-income countries where hookworm is endemic. Several of these countries, such as Brazil, China, Cuba, India, Indonesia and others, have some degree of sophistication in manufacturing health products, including vaccines.
- With genomes completed for a large number of NTD pathogens, including the agents that cause Chagas' disease, human African trypanosomiasis, leishmaniasis, leprosy, leptospirosis, LF, schistosomiasis, and trachoma, it should be theoretically possible to mine such databases in order to develop a large number of antipoverty vaccines in the coming decade.
- We have the technology in hand to develop new antipoverty vaccines, but it is financial innovation that is most needed in order to promote institutions for conducting scale-up process development, manufacturing and clinical testing and for securing global access for these new products.

Summary Points *(continued)*

- The global control and elimination of the NTDs will require mechanisms to introduce new health products, e.g., vaccines, drugs, and diagnostics, together with existing drugs, in order to create new-generation rapid-impact packages. This approach will be necessary for sustainable poverty reduction and for meeting Millennium Development Goal targets.

chapter 12

Repairing the World

There are no better grounds on which we can meet other nations and demonstrate our own concern for peace and the betterment of mankind than in a common battle against disease.
JOHN GARDNER, FORMER SECRETARY OF HEALTH, EDUCATION, AND WELFARE

...[T]ikkun olam says that, having accepted the notion that we should treat one another with respect and dignity, we come together as human beings in comity and cooperation to repair and improve the world around us.
MARIO CUOMO, FORMER GOVERNOR OF NEW YORK

While in office, and for years afterward, former New York Governor Mario Cuomo helped to popularize the Hebrew phrase *tikkun olam*, which has come to mean our moral obligation to finish the job that God began by repairing the world through social action.[1] Jewish scholars point to two 2nd-century sources for *tikkun olam*—the Aleinu prayer, now chanted at the conclusion of every Jewish prayer service, and the Mishnah, the first compendium of Jewish oral law. In the 16th century, the renowned Kabbalist Rabbi Isaac Luria expanded the use of the term. The concept of *tikkun olam* was taught to me by a mentor and cousin, Rabbi Philip Lazowski, of Beth Hillel Synagogue in Bloomfield, CT. Phil is a Holocaust survivor and the author of *Understanding Your Neighbor's Faith: What Christians and Jews Should Know about Each Other*,[2] as well as someone who has given much thought to repair. I believe that almost no other action embodies *tikkun olam* as much as the relief of human suffering through the control of the neglected tropical diseases (NTDs). In aggregate, the NTDs are the most common infections of the world's poorest people, in whom they cause chronic disability and disfigurement on a massive and, at times, almost unimaginable scale. Through their poverty-promoting impact on child development, pregnancy outcome, and worker productivity, the NTDs represent a major reason why poor people cannot lift themselves out of poverty and why the low-income countries where they live cannot economically advance. Therefore, a global assault on the NTDs through both widespread deployment of rapid-impact packages and the simultaneous development and implementation of new control tools could one day become a highly productive application of medical science and public health for repairing the world.

The control and elimination of the NTDs may also provide added global benefit in light of the underappreciated link between NTDs and human conflict. I use a definition of "conflict" proposed by Lea Berrang-Ford as "the occurrence of civil war, rebel insurgency, violent governance, political or military oppression of populations, and military combat."[3] Earlier (in chapter 7) we saw how the conflicts sweeping across the African continent, including Angola, the Democratic Republic of the Congo, the Central African Republic, and Sudan, led to a reemergence of highly lethal outbreaks of human African trypanosomiasis (HAT). In some areas of these countries, the mortality rates of sleeping sickness far exceeded those of better-known conditions, including HIV/AIDS.[3] Surveillance mapping for onchocerciasis is also incomplete in these same regions.[4] We also saw (in both chapters 5 and 7) how civil war in Sudan led to serious outbreaks of kala-azar and trachoma. The basis by which conflict has promoted the reemergence of HAT and other vector-borne NTDs has been reviewed, and at least four key determinants have been identified.[3] They include (i) economic and global effects, such as abandonment or appropriation of land, collapse of local economies, and the purging of educated and business elite, all of which lead to an interruption of public health services; (ii) a decline in specific health services, especially collapse in vector control programs; (iii) forced migration and internal displacement of populations, with resulting decreased access to health facilities, as well as land abandonment, regrowth of vegetation, and increased vector habitat; and (iv) regional insecurity and restricted access for external humanitarian support.[3]

Chris Beyer and his colleagues at Johns Hopkins University have also recently examined the relationships between specific NTDs and their unique epidemiology in conflict zones, using lymphatic filariasis (LF) in eastern Burma and Chagas' disease and leishmaniasis in Colombia as case studies.[4] In eastern Burma, ethnic minority groups have been engaged in a civil war with the military regime for decades. As a result of a government-led counterinsurgency campaign, up to 1 million Burmese have been displaced internally and another million have fled across the border into Thailand. The government of Burma has either reduced or halted diethylcarbamazine (DEC) mass drug administration efforts in the ethnic minority areas of these regions. Based on cross-sectional surveys of migrant populations coming across the Thai border, the prevalence rates of LF are now extraordinarily high (reaching 10%), while another 40% of the migrants were previously exposed to LF.[4] Today, eastern Burma has some of the highest prevalence rates of LF in Asia; an estimated 2 million cases are reported annually, but it is believed that the actual number is much higher. As Burmese immigrants find jobs in Thailand's major cities, since the appropriate mosquito vectors are present, it is anticipated that LF could reemerge in urban areas of Thailand.[4]

In Colombia, the Beyer group has also determined that the establishment of guerrilla groups together with increased cocaine drug trafficking has created an environment of extreme violence in rural areas.[4] To counter this deterioration, the Colombian government, like the Burmese government above, has dramatically escalated its military budget, often at the expense of its public health infrastructure. Colombia's vector control programs have particularly suffered, and today less than 17% of the population in areas at high risk of Chagas' disease benefits from government-led vector control programs.[4] As a result, in the northeastern part of the country near the Venezuelan border, the seroprevalence of Chagas' disease has risen to 6% or higher.[4] Similarly, those actively involved in the Colombian conflict, including military personnel and guerrillas, as well individuals who are either kidnapped or incarcerated, now frequently become infected with cutaneous leishmaniasis.[4] Military stocks of antiparasitic antimonials are now common targets for guerrilla fighters.[4]

In summary, the examples of HAT, onchocerciasis, LF, Chagas' disease, and leishmaniasis illustrate an intimate link between the NTDs and long-standing conflict. The common features of this relationship include reductions in public health control programs because of violence and a shifting of limited resources in favor of military spending and buildup. Such situations are particularly common in remote areas where guerrilla and rebel movements geographically overlap with NTDs and their vectors.[4] Also contributing to the NTD-conflict link are human migrations into areas where disease is endemic, which increase human vulnerability and often decrease access to essential medicines.[4]

Is it also possible that the NTDs not only emerge and reemerge in settings of conflict and postconflict, but that, in addition, because the NTDs themselves are destabilizing, they could ignite a series of events that culminate in conflict? Thus, just as the NTDs occur in a setting of poverty and promote poverty, could they also promote conflict? In a paper published in 2001, I showed that areas of conflict (during the last decade of the 20th century) mostly overlap geographically with areas of high infant mortality or under-age-5 child mortality.[5] Figure 12.1 shows a semiquantitative relationship between countries grouped by their under-age-5 child mortality rates and the percentage of those countries that have been engaged in armed conflict during the 1990s.[5]

In the developing regions of the world, most of the infant and under-age-5 child mortality results directly or indirectly from infectious diseases. Therefore, my interpretation of the graph is that nations with serious infectious disease problems were more likely to have been involved in armed struggles during the recent past, particularly when the under-age-5 child mortality exceeds 100 per 1,000, meaning that more than 10% of the pediatric population fails to reach its fifth birthday. Indeed, since 1990 approximately 80% of all wars have been fought in sub-Saharan Africa, Asia, and tropical regions of the Americas, especially in areas where multiple NTDs are coendemic.[5] Of interest is the observation that many of the nations with some of the worst health indicators are Islamic countries, as determined by their membership in the Organization of the Islamic Conference.[6]

These relationships do not distinguish between cause and effect, but it is highly plausible that a nation threatened by endemic infection and child morbidity and mortality would be destabilized by the large-scale effects of infection on families and civil society.[7] Michael Moodie and his colleagues at the Chemical and Biological Arms Control Institute (CBACI) have emphasized that infectious diseases and the NTDs in particular are destabilizing through (i) their impact on the agricultural workforce and their downstream effects on fields going untended, increased risks of famine, and overall lack of economic productivity; (ii) their impact on families, i.e., injuries to family breadwinners and the creation of a generation of orphans; and (iii) their impact on community governance through their disabling effects on community leaders.[7] We have seen how entire communities can be destabilized by highly endemic blindness from onchocerciasis and trachoma, widespread disability from LF and dracunculiasis, impaired child development and future productivity from hookworm infection and schistosomiasis, and widespread mortality from HAT and leishmaniasis. The demonstration of a specific link between the destabilizing effects of endemic NTDs and increased risk of conflict remains elusive, but there are sufficient connecting threads to warrant a consideration of NTD control as an element of international diplomacy.

Could we incorporate NTD control as a new element for U.S. foreign policy? Beginning in the post-Sputnik era, there has been a modest though interesting American history of linking health and diplomacy. One of the best examples occurred with the development of the live attenuated oral polio vaccine (OPV) developed by Albert Sabin during the middle and late 1950s.[5] In response to polio epidemics raging in the urban centers of both the United States and the

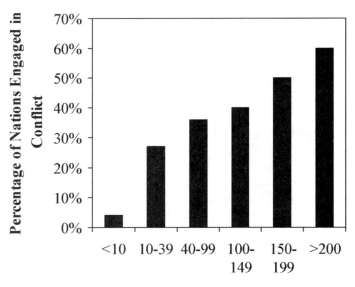

Figure 12.1 Relationship between under-age-5 childhood mortality (per 1,000) and areas of conflict during the 1990s (from Hotez, 2001b).

Soviet Union, both countries put aside their ideological differences and worked together to take Sabin's live poliovirus strains originating from his research laboratory at Cincinnati Children's Hospital to test them clinically as a vaccine in Communist Russia.[5] Many Americans are unaware that the live OPV that they received as children was licensed in the United States only after it was refined during large-scale clinical testing on tens of millions of schoolchildren in the USSR. Less than a decade later, American and Soviet microbiologists collaborated in scaling up production of a vaccine for smallpox, which led to that disease's eradication during the late 1970s.[5] Today, smallpox remains the only disease ever eradicated by humankind, a feat that occurred as a component of Cold War vaccine diplomacy![5]

During the last half of the 20th century, subsequent efforts to fully embrace vaccine diplomacy as a permanent component of U.S. foreign policy have met with mixed results. Following efforts to send medical supplies to Cuba in exchange for prisoner release after the failed Bay of Pigs invasion, the Kennedy Administration took the bold step of creating through the Department of State the U.S. Agency for International Development (USAID) and the Peace Corps.[5] Subsequently, through the advocacy of then Secretary of Health, Education, and Welfare John Gardner, the Johnson administration helped to draft legislation for the International Health Education Act.[1,5] This was an innovative proposal that would have brought medical and public health attachés to U.S. embassies worldwide. Unfortunately, the Act failed to advance through a key congressional committee and never materialized. During the 1980s and 1990s, national immunization days were a key element of cease-fires in war-torn regions of Afghanistan, Sierra Leone, and Sudan, and we saw earlier (in chapter 4) how former President Jimmy Carter was successful at brokering the guinea worm cease-fire in Sudan. In this new century, the Bush administration has launched disease control efforts for HIV/AIDS (the President's Emergency Plan for AIDS Relief [PEPFAR]), malaria (the President's Malaria Initiative [PMI]), and even an NTD Control Program for distribution of rapid-impact packages in Burkina Faso, Ghana, Mali, Niger, and Uganda (chapter 10). Each of these initiatives is administered through USAID, and they represent important first steps in infusing global disease control into U.S. foreign policy. However, for the most part, the USAID NTD Control Program and the other USAID disease control initiatives are stand-alone programs and are not truly integrated into U.S. diplomatic efforts.

Over the last decade, a handful of influential scholars of U.S. foreign policy have lamented a loss of international respect for U.S. leadership, while simultaneously pointing out the potential power of humanitarian assistance as a mechanism to restore American influence.[8] For instance, former U.S. National Security Advisor Zbigniew Brzezinski says that America must "place a higher premium on a truly shared global cause" if it is to "derive any political benefit from the cultural revolution it is unleashing worldwide" and that "the United States should treat globalization less as a gospel and more as an opportunity for the betterment of the human condition." He warns, "If American policymakers do not deliberately infuse it with politically evident moral content, focused on the alleviation of the human condition, their uncritical embrace of it could backfire."[8] Similarly, former Secretary of State Henry Kissinger states, "At the apogee of its power, the United States finds itself in an ironic position. In the face of perhaps the most profound and widespread upheavals the world has ever seen, it has failed to develop concepts relevant to the emerging realities."[8] Both Brzezinski and Kissinger, as well as Joseph Nye, Jr., the former dean of Harvard's Kennedy School of Government, are strong advocates for American humanitarian assistance, but only if it is simultaneously sustained by American domestic opinion and if it resonates with the international community and has a high probability of success.[8]

In a paper published in the *Brown Journal of World Affairs*, I argued that control of the NTDs meets all of the criteria for successful humanitarian interventions.[5] Specifically, the biblical legacy of the NTDs, together with their enormous global health impact and the relatively low cost of poverty reduction efforts, makes NTD reduction a "best buy" not only in public health but also for U.S. foreign policy.[5]

I believe that there are at least two mechanisms for pursuing NTD control in the context of our national foreign policy.

The first is in the area of research and development. The United States is known and esteemed as a world-class center of international biomedical research. Young scientists come from all over the world to study in our laboratories, and through programs sponsored by our National Institutes of Health (NIH), including the NIH's Fogarty International Center and the Tropical Medicine Research Centers (TMRC) and International Centers for Infectious Diseases Research (ICIDR) programs of the National Institute of Allergy and Infectious Diseases (NIAID), as well as the overseas laboratories of the Department of Defense and CDC in Indonesia, Peru, Kenya, and elsewhere, we have enormous capacity for training foreign scientists and fostering collaboration in overseas laboratories. These initiatives, however, are underfunded and not well linked to the exciting product development partnerships for NTD drugs and vaccines, some of which are sponsored by the Bill and Melinda Gates Foundation. We are in an excellent position to build public-private partnerships for NTDs that span government, academia, and private industry—partnerships not too different from the military-industrial complex envisioned by Vannevar Bush in his role during the 1940s and 1950s as director of the Office of Scientific Research, the umbrella organization of the Manhattan Project, as well as of the Carnegie Institution of Washington. These activities helped to transform the California universities into scientific juggernauts and overall brought scientific preeminence to the United States. Today, we could build a similar model to establish our leadership on NTDs, working in partnership with research institutes in the major innovative developing countries such as Brazil, China, India, and Indonesia. I once estimated that American vaccines had saved approximately 160 million lives, a number equivalent to all of the lives lost in global conflicts during the 20th century.[5]

At the same time, our Department of State, possibly through USAID, should work closely with the Global Network for NTD Control and other organizations to establish public-private partnerships for the widespread deployment of rapid-impact packages in the 56 countries at risk for polyparasitism and coendemic NTDs. Such an enterprise could include the appointment of a special ambassador for NTD control, just as the PEPFAR and PMI directors have ambassadorial status. The difference, however, is that an NTD equivalent of Vannevar Bush would work across the public and private sectors in order to pursue any avenue possible for NTD control.

I believe that a new government-academic-industrial enterprise devoted to NTDs offers an unprecedented new opportunity for reducing global poverty and repairing the world. We have in hand today an extraordinary toolbox of highly effective preventive chemotherapeutic drugs and the technological capacity to build a new generation of drugs and vaccines. We must heed the warning of Elie Wiesel that "Man's weakness lies not in his inability to obtain victories, but in his inability to make use of them." We have a win-win opportunity to control and eliminate humankind's major NTDs and need to act in a timely manner and with great efficiency.

What are the Neglected Tropical Diseases?

As outlined in chapter 1, the neglected tropical diseases (NTDs) are a group of chronic and disabling tropical infections. They are also poverty-promoting because of their impact on child health and development, pregnancy outcome, and worker productivity. The NTDs occur primarily in rural areas of the developing world. This book focuses primarily on a core group of 13 NTDs, including the seven most prevalent conditions—ascariasis, trichuriasis, hookworm, schistosomiasis, lymphatic filariasis, trachoma, and onchocerciasis. In addition, three important urban NTDs, namely, leptospirosis, dengue, and rabies, are addressed, as well as some important NTDs in the United States and Canada. Table 1 presents a more complete list of the NTDs.

Table 1. The NTDs[a]

Pathogen	Infection
Helminths	Ascariasis Trichuriasis Hookworm infection Strongyloidiasis Toxocariasis and larva migrans Lymphatic filariasis Onchocerciasis Loiasis Dracunculiasis Schistosomiasis Food-borne trematodiases Taeniasis-cysticercosis Echinococcosis
Protozoans	Leishmaniasis Chagas' disease Human African trypanosomiasis Amebiasis Giardiasis Balantidiasis Toxoplasmosis Trichomoniasis
Bacteria	Bartonellosis Bovine tuberculosis Buruli ulcer Leprosy Leptospirosis Relapsing fever Rheumatic fever and poststreptococcal glomerulonephritis Trachoma Treponematoses
Viruses	Dengue fever Rabies
Fungi	Mycetoma Paracoccidioidomycosis
Ectoparasites	Scabies Myiasis Tungiasis

[a]See also http://www.plosntds.org.

Notes

1. The designation of HIV/AIDS as the "plague of the 21st century" is found in Skolnik, 2007. The definition of manifesto is from Agnes (ed.), 2000, p. 874.

2. Further details of funded programs for HIV/AIDS and malaria and their relationship to the neglected tropical diseases are found in Hotez, 2006.

3. Information and table are found in Hotez et al., 2007b.

4. Further details regarding Africa's disease burden are found in Molyneux et al., 2005.

5. Information about the link between NTDs and slavery from Africa is found in Lammie et al., 2007.

6. Many of these features are excellently summarized by the World Health Organization, 2003.

7. Specific citations of ancient references on NTDs can be found in Hotez et al., 2006e.

8. Details of the estimates for deaths and DALYs resulting from the NTDs can be found in Hotez et al., 2006d.

9. Specific references for these data can be found in Hotez et al., 2007b; Hotez and Ferris, 2006; and Bleakley, 2007.

10. Interviews and qualitative analysis of patients with LF are described by Perera et al., 2007.

11. Some of the details about the relationships between stigma and health are outlined by Weiss and Ramakrishna, 2006. In addition, there are excellent descriptions of the stigmatizing aspects of NTDs in World Health Organization, 2003.

12. The three levels of neglect are described in greater detail by the World Health Organization, 2006b, p. 3. Information on the new drugs for NTDs is found in Chirac and Torreele, 2006.

13. Hunt, 2006.

14. Hotez et al., 2007b.

15. Kishore and Dhadialla, 2007.

Chapter 2

1. The Greek derivation of helminths is from Faust et al., 1970. References to the historical documentation of human ascariasis and hookworm infection are found in Cox, 2002; Grove, 1990; and Sherman, 2006, p. 349–352.

2. Prevalence numbers are from Bethony et al., 2006.

3. The impact of STHs on child growth and development and cognition is summarized (with references) by Bethony et al., 2006, and Crompton and Nesheim, 2002. The Crompton and Nesheim reference also describes the nutritional basis of these deficits. Photos in Fig. 2.1 taken by NPR's Brigid McCarthy were originally posted on NPR.org's weekend Edition Saturday page on October 29, 2005, and are used with the permission of NPR.

4. The results of the nationwide parasite survey are summarized by Hotez et al., 1997. The survey was later repeated (but on a smaller scale) between 2002 and 2004 and demonstrated that the incidence had since decreased dramatically in areas of economic development. The new Chinese prevalence numbers are reported by Bethony et al., 2006.

5. These observations are summarized by Hotez, 2002b.

6. These observations are reported by Fenghua et al., 1998.

7. From de Silva et al., 2003. The figure was also reproduced with permission by Hotez et al., 2005.

8. Factors underlying the relationship between STH infection and poverty are described by Raso et al., 2005; Holland et al., 1988; and Hotez, 2007a.

9. The exact mechanisms by which STHs impair growth and development are still poorly understood. An excellent review of the literature is found in Crompton and Nesheim, 2002.

10. Miguel and Kremer, 2003.

11. The link between STHs and impaired cognition and memory has been studied extensively by D. A. P. Bundy and his colleagues. Two important papers include Nokes et al., 1992, and Sakti et al., 1999. However, the mechanisms by which worms impair cognition and memory are not well understood.

12. Bleakley, 2007. Some of the data are also in Bleakley, 2006.

13. Original maps of the distribution of all three STH infections can be found in de Silva et al., 2003.

14. An excellent historical account of hookworm in the United States is found in Ettling, 1981. A more global perspective can be found in Farley, 2004.

15. Humphreys, 2001.

16. A summary of the impact of sanitation and health education on STH infections is found in Asaolu and Ofoezie, 2003. A study showing the absence of a relationship between wearing shoes and avoiding hookworm infection is found in Bethony et al., 2002.

17. Descriptions of the hookworm life cycle and the clinical manifestations of hookworm are found in Hotez et al., 2005, and Hotez et al., 2004.

18. Studies showing a high hookworm prevalence and intensity in coastal regions (regions with sandy soils) are in Mabaso et al., 2003, and Mabaso et al., 2004.

19. The biochemical mechanism by which hookworms digest blood is described by Williamson et al., 2004.

20. Some of these calculations can be found in Stoltzfus et al., 1997a, and Stoltzfus et al., 1997b. They are summarized by Crompton, 2000, and Crompton and Nesheim, 2002.

21. The global importance of hookworm in pregnancy is highlighted by Bundy et al., 1995, and Christian et al., 2004.

22. Data are summarized by Hotez et al., 2006d.

23. Information on the control of STH infections through deworming is summarized by Albonico et al., 2006; Brooker et al., 2004; and Crompton and Nesheim, 2002. Some investigators consider the improvements in child cognition that result from deworming to be marginal or controversial; see Dickson et al., 2000.

24. Hotez et al., 2006c; World Bank, 2003.

25. Savioli et al., 1992.

26. Estimates of the scope of global deworming are in Horton, 2003.

27. This information is summarized by Brooker et al., 2004.

28. This information is summarized by Hotez et al., 2006b.

Chapter 3

1. Estimates are from Steinmann et al., 2006.

2. Historical accounts of schistosomiasis are found in Hulse, 1971; Hotez et al., 2006e; Cox, 2002; Fenwick et al., 2006; and Grove, 1990.

3. Ross et al., 2007.

4. This incident is described by Kernan, 1959. Because the article is not easy to find, readers may also read a summary of this information in Farley, 1991.

5. Information is contained in Lampton, 1974.

6. Information is found in Horn, 1969; Hotez, 2002b; Utzinger et al., 2005; and Farley, 1991, p. 201–215.

7. Wei, 1958, quoted by Farley, 1991, p. 206.

8. The impact of dam construction projects on the emergence of human schistosomiasis is described by Fenwick, 2006, and Hotez et al., 1997.

9. Farley, 1991, p. 45–54, 188–200.

10. Information is contained in Fenwick et al., 2006.

11. Hotez et al., 2006c.

12. Information about the link between schistosomiasis and other NTDs and slavery from Africa is found in Lammie et al., 2007.

13. Gryseels et al., 2006.

14. The morbid effects of long-standing schistosomiasis are described by King et al., 2005.

15. Van der Werf et al., 2003.

16. Kjetland et al., 2006.

17. Fenwick and Webster, 2006.

18. Papers on schistosomiasis and hookworm coinfections include Raso et al., 2006, and Fleming et al., 2006.

19. Kabatereine et al., 2006.

20. King et al., 2006.

21. Utzinger et al., 2001.

22. Capron et al., 2005.

Chapter 4

1. Historical accounts of LF and dracunculiasis are found in Cox, 2002, and Hotez et al., 2006a. Quote from *Tales of the South Pacific* from *Time*, 1962.

2. Information on the prevalence of LF and the estimates that approximately 1 billion people in these developing regions are at risk of acquiring the disease are found in Ottesen, 2006.

3. These numbers are quoted from Rajan, 2005.

4. Today, diagnosing LF can be done by sampling the blood at any time of the day and chemically detecting the presence of *W. bancrofti* antigen through use of a card known as an ICT card or test, the development of which was pioneered by Gary Weil at Washington University in St. Louis.

5. This is discussed by Babu et al., 2006, and Nutman and Kumaraswami, 2001.

6. A good description of the pathologic sequence of events in patients with LF is found in Addiss and Brady, 2007.

7. There are several excellent published clinical descriptions of LF and elephantiasis. The one that I like best is by Simonsen, 2002.

8.   Figures are from Michael et al., 1996.

9.   The productivity losses from LF are described by Perera et al., 2007, and Global Alliance to Eliminate Lymphatic Filariasis, 2004.

10. The economic impact of LF has been reported in at least three papers: Ramaiah et al., 2000a; Ramaiah et al., 2000b; and Babu, 2002.

11. Some of the senior Hawking's work is summarized by Hawking et al., 1950; Hawking, 1955; and Hawking, 1958.

12. Coggeshall, 1945; quoted by Rajan, 2005.

13. Kessel et al., 1953.

14. Hawking and Marques, 1967.

15. Zhong and Zhen, 1991.

16. Houston, 2000.

17. Ramzy et al., 2006.

18. Ichimori et al., 2007.

19. Ottesen, 2006.

20. Fiftieth World Health Assembly, 1997b.

21. Global guinea worm eradication efforts are summarized by Hopkins et al., 2005, and Ruiz-Tiben and Hopkins, 2006.

22. Cairncross et al., 2002.

23. The account here of the modern history of guinea worm eradication is summarized from Levine et al., 2004, p. 91–104. The book contains a number of interesting histories of successes in NTD control and in global health.

24. World Health Organization, 2008g.

25. Fiftieth World Health Assembly, 1997a.

26. Carter Center, 2006.

27. Hopkins and Withers, 2002.

28. The economic figures are from Kim et al., 1997, and are quoted in note 21 (Ruiz-Tiben and Hopkins, 2006).

29. McNeil, 2006, and Barry, 2006.

Chapter 5

1.   Quote from Robert McNamara in International Bank for Reconstruction and Development, 2004.

2.   Estimates are from Dandona and Dandona, 2006. Their numbers are higher than the WHO figures, which suggest that 161 million people have visual impairments and 37 million people are blind. Blindness is defined as visual acuity of less than 3/60 in the better eye.

3. In developing countries, the leading causes of pediatric blindness are vitamin A deficiency, congenital cataract, and ophthalmia neonatorum, an infectious disease; in adults the leading causes of blindness are cataract, trachoma, and chronic glaucoma (McGavin, 2002).

4. Papers on infectious and other causes of blindness as a consequence of the war are found in Buchan, 2006, and Ngondi et al., 2006.

5. The WHO Prevention of Blindness (PBL) team works with member states to prevent blindness and restore sight. Its global target is to reduce the prevalence of blindness to less than 0.5% in all countries or less than 1% in any particular country. World Health Organization, 2008f.

6. Courtright et al., 1997.

7. Basanez et al., 2006.

8. World Health Organization, 1995.

9. Boatin and Richard, 2006.

10. Information about the clinical descriptions of onchocerciasis is from Simonsen, 2002.

11. A description of these *Wolbachia* bacterial endoparasites can be found in Taylor et al., 2005.

12. Kale, 1998.

13. Information is contained in Amazigo et al., 2006.

14. Papers on stigma and OSD include Amazigo and Obikeze, 1992, and Vlassoff et al., 2000.

15. The story of Robert McNamara's interest in onchocerciasis can be found in Cobb, 2001.

16. Excellent descriptions of the modern history of programs for onchocerciasis control can be found in Boatin and Richard, 2006, and Levine et al., 2004, p. 54–64.

17. The history of ivermectin development can be found in Campbell, 1991, and Geary, 2005.

18. Information about APOC and OEPA can be found at African Programme for Onchocerciasis Control, 2005, and World Health Organization, 2008d.

19. Up to a ninefold increase in bed net distribution was observed in Nigeria. Blackburn et al., 2006.

20. An important paper on possible emerging ivermectin resistance and an accompanying commentary can be found in Osei-Atweneboana et al., 2007, and Hotez, 2007b.

21. General papers on trachoma and blindness in developing countries include Kasi et al., 2004, and Buchan, 2006.

22. The economic burden estimates are in Frick et al., 2003b, and Frick et al., 2003a.

23. Allen and Semba, 2002.

24. Rearwin et al., 1997.

25. Information on the clinical and epidemiological description of trachoma is from McGavin, 2002.

26. An excellent description of the formation of ITI and the use of azithromycin for the control of trachoma in Morocco and elsewhere can be found in Levine et al., 2004, p. 83–89; International Trachoma Initiative, 2008; and International Trachoma Initiative, 2006.

27. Kumaresan, 2005.

Chapter 6

1. The first quotation is from Stienstra et al., 2002. The quotation in Leviticus is discussed by Guzik, 2004.

2. Plorde, 2004.

3. The five elements of DOTS include political commitment, case detection, standardized treatment with supervision, an effective drug supply and management system, and a monitoring and evaluation system (World Health Organization, 2008e).

4. Clancey et al., 1962.

5. Johnson et al., 2005.

6. New information on the clinical and epidemiological aspects of Buruli ulcer is from Wansbrough-Jones and Phillips, 2006, and Sizaire, 2006.

7. Detailed information about the mycolactone toxin and the *M. ulcerans* genes that encode it can be found in George et al., 1999, and Stinear et al., 2004.

8. Papers on the plasmids expressing *M. ulcerans* mycolactone toxin-associated genes are found in Stinear et al., 2004, and are summarized by Townsend, 2004.

9. The role of aquatic insects in the transmission of Buruli ulcer was first suggested in 1999 as described by Portaels et al., 1999. A more recent summary of the subsequent literature is found in Silva et al., 2007.

10. A summary of the antipoverty vaccines is provided by Hotez and Ferris, 2006.

11. A good historical overview of leprosy can be found in Roueché, 1986, p. 68–86. Berton Roueché wrote about medical mysteries as part of the "Annals of Medicine" feature in the *New Yorker* magazine for more than 40 years. He died in 1994 at the age of 83. An account of his life can be found in Lerner, 2005.

12. Another very good historical account is found in chapter 14 of Sherman, 2006, p. 303–311.

13. This theory was advanced by Donoghue et al., 2005.

14. The history of the National Leprosarium in Carville is told by Furman, 1973, and Gaudet, 2004.

15. World Health Organization, 2008c.

16. Clinical information on leprosy is from Leprosy Group, WHO, 2002.

17. Tsutsumi et al., 2007.

18. Rinaldi, 2005.

19. Lockwood and Suneetha, 2005.

20. Cole et al., 2001.

21. Lockwood, 2004.

Chapter 7

1. The reemergence of HAT and leishmaniasis as a result of conflict in Africa is described by Anonymous, 1997; Ritmeijer and Davidson, 2003; and Collin et al., 2006.

2. Information on the epidemiology and clinical features of HAT is from Burri and Brun, 2002; Pepin and Meda, 2001; and Fèvre et al., 2006.

3. Information is from Sherman, 2006, p. 325–330.

4. The lytic properties of HDL against trypanosomes were discovered in the 1970s by Mary ("Miki") Rifkin, then at The Rockefeller University. A recent review of this phenomenon is in Pays et al., 2006.

5. The term variable surface glycoproteins or "VSGs" is used to describe the antigens responsible for variation. The cellular and molecular mechanisms of antigenic variation in trypanosomes were first described in the 1970s by Keith Vickerman, working at the University of Glasgow, and George Cross, then at Cambridge University and now at The Rockefeller University. A recent review of this phenomenon can be found in Pays et al., 2004.

6. Historical accounts of HAT and other kinetoplastid infections are in Cox, 2004; Sherman, 2006; and Hoppe, 2003. The quotation at the opening of this chapter is from Conrad, 1902, p. 31–32.

7. Both the Liverpool School of Tropical Medicine and the London School of Tropical Medicine were established in 1899. The London School was renamed the London School of Hygiene in Tropical Medicine coinciding with funding from the Rockefeller Foundation in 1924. An account of the Liverpool School can be found in Power, 1999. An account of the London School can be found in Haynes, 2001.

8. Paul Ehrlich defined chemotherapy as "the use of drugs to injure an invading organism without injury to the host." This information is contained in Riethmiller, 2005. Work on the development of tryparsamide by Louise Pearce at the Rockefeller Institute for Medical Research is described by Pearce, 1921.

9. A description of PTRE and other neurologic sequelae of HAT in the central nervous system is in Kennedy, 2006.

10. The summary paper on the *T. brucei* genome is in Berriman et al., 2005. The activities of DNDi are described by Pecoul, 2004.

11. High-throughput screening for antitrypanosomal drugs is described by McKerrow, 2005.

12. Bisser et al., 2007, and Pepin, 2007.

13. The two major approaches for the control of HAT are described by Fèvre et al., 2006.

14. A more detailed account of the career of Eugene Jamot can be found in Naval and Overseas Health Association, 2001–2008.

15. The story of the reemergence of human trypanosomiasis in Angola is told by Stanghellini and Josenando, 2001, and Abel et al., 2004.

16. Odiit et al., 2004.

17. Welburn et al., 2006.

18. I credit the phrase "conflict and contagion" to Michael Moody, who heads the Chemical and Biological Arms Control Institute (CBACI), a Washington, DC-based policy think tank.

19. Excellent historical descriptions of Carlos Chagas and his contributions to medical science are in Lewinsohn, 2003, and Sá, 2005.

20. Figure according to WHO Expert Committee on the Control of Chagas Disease, 2002, p. i–vi, 1–109, back cover.

21. The vector control programs for Chagas' disease are described by Yamagata and Nakagawa, 2006.

22. The account from Darwin is found in Sá, 2005. Darwin's possible affliction with Chagas' disease is described by Bernstein, 1984.

23. The molecular and cellular mechanisms by which *T. cruzi* invades cells and then replicates are elegantly described by Andrade and Andrews, 2005.

24. Information on the clinical aspects of Chagas' disease is from Miles, 2002, and Teixeira et al., 2006b.

25. Information on the long-term pathogenesis of cardiomyopathy is found in Marin-Neto et al., 2007. A classical description of Chagas' pathology by Fritz Koberle is found in Koberle, 1968.

26. The publication of the *T. cruzi* genome is in El-Sayed et al., 2005.

27. Schofield et al., 2006.

28. Based on information contained in Alvar et al., 2006a.

29. Information on the clinical, epidemiological, and life cycle aspects of CL and VL is from Murray et al., 2005.

30. The stigmatizing and poverty-promoting aspects of leishmaniasis are described by Alvar et al., 2006b.

31. An account of the Sudanese leishmaniasis epidemic is in Zijlstra and El-Hassan, 2001.

32. The role of sandflies in the transmission of leishmaniasis was not conclusively demonstrated until 1941, by Saul Adler and his colleague M. Ber. Adler became a

professor at Hebrew University and was considered one of the founding fathers of modern parasitology in Israel.

33. Institute for One World Health, 2008.

Chapter 8

1. Information is contained in Erlanger et al., 2005, and Utzinger and Keiser, 2006.

2. Information is found in Gubler et al., 2001.

3. A good overview of leptospirosis is found in Bharti et al., 2003, and McBride et al., 2005.

4. A description of urban leptospirosis in the United States and elsewhere is found in Vinetz et al., 1996.

5. Scott and Coleman, 2002.

6. John, 2005.

7. Cachay and Vinetz, 2005.

8. A description of dengue fever in the favelas can be found in Heukelbach et al., 2001.

9. The reemergence of dengue in South America and elsewhere is described by Gubler and Clark, 1995.

10. World Health Organization, 2008h.

11. Malavige et al., 2004.

12. Nimmannitya, 2002.

13. Scott Halstead, formerly of the Rockefeller Foundation and founding director of the Pediatric Dengue Vaccine Initiative, is largely credited with the sequential infection hypothesis of DHF. It is summarized by Halstead, 1981.

14. WHO's DengueNET activities are described by World Health Organization, 2008a.

15. Singapore's efforts to control dengue were reported by Arnold, 2007.

16. Copepod control in Vietnam is described by Kay et al., 2002.

17. Information on hydrophobia and other features of clinical rabies is from Warrell, 2002.

18. The historical accounts are summarized in note 13 and by Theodorides, 1986. The statement on rabies in the Babylon Codex is in World Health Organization, 2008b. The quotation from it at the beginning of the chapter is found in chapter 39, "Rhabdoviridae: History," p. 1363, in Knipe and Hawley, 2007.

19. The global burden of human rabies is described by Wyatt, 2007, and Coleman et al., 2004.

20. An assessment of India's disease burden can be found online in Sudarshan, 2005.

21. The economic impact of rabies is summarized by Meltzer and Rupprecht, 1998.

22. Dinh, 2001.

23. An excellent description of the sequence of pathologic events leading to clinical rabies is in Warrell and Warrell, 2004.

24. Information is found in United Nations Population Fund, 2007. The issue was also reported by Dugger, 2007.

25. Information is found in United Nations Human Settlements Programme, 2003.

Chapter 9

1. The socioeconomic impact of tropical diseases in the American South is a topic of works by the medical historian Margaret Humphreys, including Humphreys, 2001, and Martin and Humphreys, 2006. Also, the economist Hoyt Bleakley has written about the impact of hookworm in Bleakley, 2007.

2. The finding that 36.5 million Americans live in poverty is from the U.S. Census Bureau, 2007.

3. Some papers on the prevalence of hookworm in the United States during the last half of the 20th century include Henderson, 1957; Farmer, 1983; Arnold, 1949; Disalvo and Melonas, 1970; Sargent et al., 1972; and Martin, 1972.

4. The high prevalence of ascariasis and trichuriasis among Cherokee Indian schoolchildren was reported by Healy et al., 1969.

5. Data are found in Chorazy and Richardson, 2005.

6. A summary of covert toxocariasis is provided by Sharghi et al., 2000.

7. Toxocariasis infection rates during the 1970s are found in Hermann et al., 1985.

8. The Connecticut study is reported by Sharghi et al., 2001.

9. The New York study is reported by Marmor et al., 1987.

10. Busse and Mitchell, 2007.

11. The relationship between toxocariasis and asthma is found in Buijs et al., 1997, and Kuk et al., 2006.

12. The table used for calculations as follows (extrapolated from resident population of major U.S. cities by race and Hispanic origins, 2000) is found in Wright (ed.), 2006, p. 243–245.

13. Data are found in Siddiqui and Berk, 2001.

14. Centers for Disease Control and Prevention, 2002.

15. Del La Garza et al., 2005.

16. White and Atmar, 2002.

17. Wallin and Kurtzke, 2004.

18. DeGiorgio et al., 2005a, and DeGiorgio et al., 2005b. Cysticercosis is also a significant cause of death, responsible for 221 deaths between 1990 and 2002 (Sorvillo et al., 2007). See also Ong et al., 2002.

19. Jones et al., 2003.

20. Data on the U.S. disease burden of congenital toxoplasmosis are found in Lopez et al., 2000.

21. McLeod et al., 2006.

22. Kim, 2006.

23. Hlvasa et al., 2005.

24. Information about leishmaniasis and Chagas' disease in Texas and elsewhere can be found in Maloney et al., 2002; Jacobson, 2007; Willard et al., 2005; Weina et al., 2004; Enserink, 2000; and Hanford et al., 2007.

25. Information about trachoma on the Navajo Reservation is in Rearwin et al., 1997, and Ludlam, 1978.

26. The impact of climate change on vector- and rodent-borne diseases and dengue and lepstospirosis in the United States is summarized by Gubler et al., 2001; Vinetz et al., 1996; and the Centers for Disease Control and Prevention, 2005.

27. Proulx et al., 2002.

28. The clinical syndrome caused by *T. s. nativa* was described first by J. D. MacLean and his associates at the Centre for Tropical Diseases of McGill University. See MacLean et al., 1992, and MacLean et al., 1989.

29. McDonald et al., 1990.

30. Rausch, 2003.

31. Wilson et al., 1995.

32. Information about onchocerciasis in Mexico is from the World Health Organization, 2006c.

33. Information about hookworm and other soil-transmitted helminth infections in Mexico is from Brentlinger et al., 2003, and Quihui-Cota et al., 2004.

34. Information about cutaneous leishmaniasis in Chiapas State as well as in the Yucatan is found in Flisser et al., 2002; Andrade-Narvaez et al., 2001; and Rebollar-Tellez et al., 2005.

35. An interesting debate about the extent of Chagas' disease in Mexico is in the following Lancet correspondence: Attaran, 2006, and Conyer, 2006.

36. Information on the prevalence of NTDs in the Caribbean comes from the following sources: for schistosomiasis, see Chitsulo et al., 2000, which cites 15,000 cases of schistosomiasis in Puerto Rico. However, a more recent reference (Hillyer, 2005) suggests that schistosomiasis is nearing elimination on the island. On LF, one source is available. See estimates in 2006, from the World Health Organization, 2006a. For dengue (2006 data only; only countries with more than 30 cases shown), see Pan American Health Organization, 2007.

37. Information on the prevalence of soil-transmitted helminth infections in the Caribbean is summarized by Ehrenberg, 2002.

38. Information about the link between NTDs and slavery from Africa is found in Lammie et al., 2007.

Chapter 10

1. Based on information from Hotez et al., 2006d, and Hotez et al., 2007b.

2. A paper pointing out the importance of incorporating the chronic effects of schistosomiasis and other NTDs into DALY estimates can be found in King et al., 2005. See also King, 2007.

3. Information is summarized by Hotez and Ferris, 2006, and Hotez et al., 2007b.

4. A summary of the World Health Assembly resolutions on NTDs is found in Brady et al., 2006. Table 10.2 is based on information contained in Brady et al., 2006, and Hotez et al., 2007b. The major target populations have a number of important exceptions (sometimes including pregnant or lactating women or very young children) that are detailed in these two references.

5. Statistical information on Cote d'Ivoire is found in Wright (ed.), 2006.

6. Information on polyparasitism in Cote d'Ivoire, Brazil, and elsewhere is found in Raso et al., 2004; Raso et al., 2006; Fleming et al., 2006; and McKenzie, 2005.

7. Information is found in Brooker and Utzinger, 2007.

8. Combined disease burden of the NTDs is found in Hotez et al., 2006d, and Hotez, et al., 2007b.

9. The rationale of the rapid-impact package is in Molyneux et al., 2005. The definition of the rapid-impact package is in Hotez et al., 2007b.

10. Information on the health and cognitive impact of the rapid-impact package is found in Hotez et al., 2006d.

11. Information is in Hotez et al., 2006d.

12. Information on the global impact of anemia is in Zimmermann and Hurrell, 2007.

13. Information on the impact of deworming on anemia rates in children and in pregnant women is in Hotez et al., 2006d; Torlesse and Hodges, 2000; and Christian et al., 2004.

14. Information on the impact of deworming and anemia reduction on education and economic development is in Miguel and Kremer, 2003; World Bank, 2003; and Bleakley, 2007.

15. The costs of integrated NTD control are provided by Fenwick et al., 2005; Brady et al., 2006; and Hotez et al., 2007b.

16. The US$3 billion annual estimate for malaria control in Africa is from Teklehaimanot et al., 2007, and Sachs and Hotez, 2006. Estimates of dollars per

DALY averted are in Laxminarayan et al., 2006. A further comparison of deworming with major control measures for malaria, tuberculosis, and HIV/AIDS reveals that insecticide-treated nets for malaria cost US$2 to US$24 per DALY averted, direct observed treatment for tuberculosis costs US$5 to US$35 per DALY averted, and antiretroviral therapy costs US$350 to US$500 per DALY averted.

17. Canning, 2006.

18. World Health Organization, 2006d.

19. Information about the Global Network and its partners is in Hotez et al., 2007b. The URL for the Global Network is at http://www.sabin.org/gnntdc.

20. Kristof, 2007.

21. The challenges of integration are detailed by Hotez et al., 2007a, and Hotez et al., 2007b.

22. The use of GIS/RS in NTD mapping and control is described by Brooker et al., 2006a; Brooker et al., 2002; and Brooker, 2002.

23. Studies of the integration of insecticide-treated net distribution with MDA are described by Blackburn et al., 2006.

24. The geographic overlap between malaria and hookworm infection is in Brooker et al., 2006b.

25. Information is from Brooker et al., 2007.

26. The impact of hookworm infection and malaria on pregnancy in Africa is described by Crompton, 2000; Guyatt and Snow, 2004; and Torlesse and Hodges, 2000.

27. The "perfect storm" of anemia and the agricultural anemias are described by Hotez et al., 2006d, and Fleming, 1994.

28. The synergistic effects between NTDs and malaria are summarized by Druilhe et al., 2005.

29. The entry points between NTD and malaria control are summarized by Hotez et al., 2006d, and Brooker et al., 2007. Relevant specific papers on IPT for malaria include Greenwood, 2006, and Ntab et al., 2007.

30. Sachs and Hotez, 2006.

31. The impact of NTDs on the HIV/AIDS epidemic is described by the following papers: Borkow and Bentwich, 2006; Secor, 2006; Kjetland et al., 2006; and Gallagher et al., 2005.

Chapter 11

1. The impact of malaria control on economic development in southern Europe is described by Gallup and Sachs, 2001.

2. The history of drug resistance in global malaria eradication efforts is described by Harrison, 1978, and Hotez, 2004.

3. Some of the mathematical concepts regarding drug resistance, pathogen transmission, and population genetics are in Anderson, 1999, and Austin et al., 1997.

4. Drug resistance and its impact on livestock production are described by Conder and Campbell, 1995.

5. Detection of the benzimidazole-resistant phenotype in *W. bancrofti* and the evidence for resistance to benzimidazole by hookworms are described or summarized by Prichard, 2007; Schwab et al., 2007; Schwab et al., 2005; Bennet and Guyatt, 2000; Albonico et al., 2004b; Albonico et al., 2003; Albonico et al., 2004a; and Albonico et al., 2006.

6. Evidence for emerging ivermectin resistance against *Onchocerca volvulus* is found in Osei-Atweneboana et al., 2007, and Hotez, 2007b.

7. Prichard, 2007.

8. Descriptions of tribendimidine, moxidectin, and anti-*Wolbachia* therapies as possible drugs for human helminth infections are found in Xiao et al., 2005; Cotreau et al., 2003; Taylor et al., 2005; and Kaminsky et al., 2008.

9. Some earlier-stage anthelmintic drug development projects are described by Greenwood et al., 2005; Tripathi et al., 2006; Ribeiro-dos-Santos et al., 2006; and Shuhua et al., 2000.

10. Information is from Chirac and Torreele, 2006.

11. Novartis has established an innovative Institute for Tropical Diseases (Novartis Institute for Tropical Diseases) in order to discover small molecules for the treatment of dengue and tuberculosis (http://www.nitd.novartis.com).

12. Moran, 2005.

13. Kremer and Glennerster, 2004, and Brownback, 2007.

14. The comparison of the genomes for the two human trypanosomes and leishmania is in El Sayed et al., 2005.

15. The PDP/public-private partnership activities for developing new drugs to combat kinetoplastid infections are described by Renslo and McKerrow, 2006; Croft et al., 2005; Croft et al., 2006; Mathis et al., 2006; and Hotez et al., 2007b.

16. Hotez and Ferris, 2006.

17. Summaries of PDP efforts to develop vaccines for schistosomiasis, leishmaniasis, hookworm infection, dengue, and nagana are found in Capron et al., 2005; Coler and Reed, 2005; Hotez et al., 2006b; Diemert et al., 2008; Edelman, 2007; and Lubega et al., 2002.

18. Bergquist et al., 2005.

19. Steps required to produce a vaccine in the nonprofit sector are described by Bottazzi et al., 2006.

20. The efforts of HHVI are described by Goozner, 2007, and Hathaway, 2007.

21. The problems of vaccine global access are described by Mahoney and Maynard, 1999, and Mahoney et al., 2007.

22. Morel et al., 2005.

Chapter 12

1. The phrase *tikkun olam* appears in many of Mario Cuomo's writings and speeches. The quotation at the beginning of the chapter is found in Pew Forum on Religion & Public Life, 2002. The Gardner quotation is found in Carey, 1970.

2. Lazowski's books include Lazowski, 2004.

3. The role of conflict and its impact on HAT are articulated by Berrang-Ford, 2007.

4. The role of conflict and its impact on LF and Chagas' disease transmission are described by Beyer et al., 2007.

5. I have explored the relationship between conflict and infectious diseases in several articles, including Hotez, 2001a; Hotez, 2001b; Hotez, 2006; and Broder et al., 2002.

6. The relationship between conflict and infection with regard to the Organization of the Islamic Conference is explored in Hotez, 2002a.

7. The destabilizing effects of ill health and security are nicely articulated by Schneider and Moodie, 2002, and Guha-Sapir and van Panhuis, 2002.

8. Quotations and citations are found in Kissinger, 2001; Brzezinski, 2004; and Nye, 1999. These quotations are also found in Hotez, 2001b; Hotez, 2006; and Hotez, 2002a.

References

Abel, P. M., G. Kiala, V. Loa, M. Behrend, J. Musolf, H. Fleischmann, J. Theophile, S. Krishna, and A. Stich. 2004. Retaking sleeping sickness control in Angola. *Trop. Med. Int. Health* **9:**141–148.

Addiss, D. G., and M. A. Brady. 2007. Morbidity management of the Global Programme to Eliminate Lymphatic Filariasis: a review of the scientific literature. *Filaria J.* **6:**2.

African Programme for Onchocerciasis Control. 2005. The African Programme for Onchocerciasis Control (APOC). African Programme for Onchocerciasis Control, Dugadougov, Burkina Faso. http://www.apoc.bf/en. Accessed 9 February 2008.

Agnes, M. (ed.). 2000. *Webster's New World College Dictionary*, 4th ed., p. 874. Wiley, New York, NY.

Albonico, M., Q. Bickle, M. Ramsan, A. Montresor, L. Savioli, and M. Taylor. 2003. Efficacy of mebendazole and levamisole alone or in combination against intestinal nematode infections after repeated targeted mebendazole treatment in Zanzibar. *Bull. W. H. O.* **81:**343–352.

Albonico, M., D. Engels, and L. Savioli. 2004a. Monitoring drug efficacy and early detection of drug resistance in human soil-transmitted nematodes: a pressing public health agenda for helminth control. *Int. J. Parasitol.* **34:**1205–1210.

Albonico, M., A. Montresor, D. W. T. Crompton, and L. Savioli. 2006. Intervention for the control of soil-transmitted helminthiasis in the community. *Adv. Parasitol.* **61:**311–348.

Albonico, M., V. Wright, and O. Bickle. 2004b. Molecular analysis of the beta-tubulin gene of human hookworms as a basis for possible benzimidazole resistance on Pemba Island. *Mol. Biochem. Parasitol.* **134:**281–284.

Allen, S. K., and R. D. Semba. 2002. The trachoma menace in the United States, 1897–1960. *Surv. Ophthalmol.* **47:**500–509.

Alvar, J., S. Croft, and P. Olliaro. 2006a. Chemotherapy in the treatment and control of leishmaniasis. *Adv. Parasitol.* **61:**223–274.

Alvar, J., S. Yactayo, and C. Bern. 2006b. Leishmaniasis and poverty. *Trends Parasitol.* **22:**552–557.

Amazigo, U., M. Noma, J. Bump, B. Benton, B. Liese, L. Yameogo, H. Zoure, and A. Seketeli. 2006. Onchocerciasis, p. 215–222. *In* D. T. Jamison, R. G. Feachem, M. W. Makgoba, E. R. Bos, F. K. Bingana, K. J. Hofman, and K. O. Rogo (ed.), *Disease and Mortality in Sub-Saharan Africa*, 2nd ed. World Bank, Washington, DC.

Amazigo, U. O., and D. S. Obikeze. 1992. Socio-cultural factors associated with the prevalence and intensity of onchocerciasis and onchodermatitis among adolescent girls in rural Nigeria. WHO/TDR Discussion Paper. World Health Organization, Geneva, Switzerland.

Anderson, R. M. 1999. The pandemic of antibiotic resistance. *Nat. Med.* **5:**147–149.

Andrade, L. O., and N. W. Andrews. 2005. The *Trypanosoma cruzi*-host-cell interplay: location, invasion, retention. *Nat. Rev. Microbiol.* **3:**819–823.

Andrade-Narvaez, F. J., A. Vargas-Gonzalez, S. B. Canto-Lara, and A. G. Damian-Centeno. 2001. Clinical picture of cutaneous leishmaniasis due to Leishmania (Leishmania) mexicana in the Yucatan peninsula. *Mem. Inst. Oswaldo Cruz* **96:**163–167.

Anonymous. 1997. Trypanosomiasis re-emerges under cover of war. *Afr. Health* **19**:3.

Arnold, J. H. 1949. The public health problems of hookworm disease in South Carolina. *J. S. C. Med. Assoc.* **45**:367–369.

Arnold, W. 2007. Mosquitoes have the edge in Singapore's dengue war. *N. Y. Times* **2007**:(12 June).

Asaolu, S. O., and I. E. Ofoezie. 2003. The role of health education and sanitation in the control of helminth infections. *Acta Tropica* **86**:283–294.

Attaran, A. 2006. Chagas disease in Mexico. *Lancet* **368**:1768.

Austin, D. J., M. Kakehashi, and R. M. Anderson. 1997. The transmission dynamics of antibiotic-resistant bacteria: the relationship between resistance in commensal organisms and antibiotic consumption. *Proc. Biol. Sci.* **264**:1629–1638.

Babu, B. V., A. N. Nayak, A. S. Acharya, P. K. Jangid, and G. Mallick. 2002. The economic loss due to treatment costs and work loss to individuals with chronic lymphatic filariasis in rural communities of Orissa, India. *Acta Tropica* **82**:31–38.

Babu, S., C. P. Blauvelt, V. Kumaraswami, and T. B. Nutman. 2006. Regulatory networks induced by live parasites impair both Th1 and Th2 pathways in patent lymphatic filariasis: implications for parasite persistence. *J. Immunol.* **176**:3248–3256.

Barry, M. 2006. Slaying little dragons: lessons from the dracunculiasis eradication program. *Am. J. Trop. Med. Hyg.* **75**:1–2.

Basanez, M. G., S. D. S. Pion, T. S. Churcher, L. P. Breitling, M. P. Little, and M. Boussinesq. 2006. River blindness: a success story under threat? *PLoS Med.* **3**:1454–1460 (e371).

Bennet, A., and H. Guyatt. 2000. Reducing intestinal nematode infection: efficacy of albendazole and mebendazole. *Parasitol. Today* **2**:71–74.

Bergquist, N. R., L. R. Leonardo, and G. F. Mitchell. 2005. Vaccine-linked chemotherapy: can schistosomiasis control benefit from an integrated approach? *Trends Parasitol.* **21**:112–117.

Bernstein, R. E. 1984. Darwin's illness: Chagas' disease resurgens. *J. R. Soc. Med.* **77**:608–609.

Berrang-Ford, L. 2007. Civil conflict and sleeping sickness in Africa in general and Uganda in particular. *Confl. Health* **1**:6.

Berriman, M., E. Ghedin, C. Hertz-Fowler, et al. 2005. The genome of the African trypanosome Trypanosoma brucei. *Science* **309**:416–422.

Bethony, J., S. Brooker, M. Albonico, S. F. Geiger, A. Loukas, D. Diemert, and P. J. Hotez. 2006. Soil-transmitted helminth infections: ascariasis, trichuriasis, and hookworm. *Lancet* **367**:1521–1532.

Bethony, J., J. Chen, S. Lin, S. Xiao, B. Zhan, S. Li, H. Xue, F. Xing, D. Humphries, W. Yan, G. Chen, V. Foster, J. M. Hawdon, and P. J. Hotez. 2002. Emerging patterns of hookworm infection: influence of aging on the intensity of Necator infection in Hainan Province, People's Republic of China. *Clin. Infect. Dis.* **35**:1336–1344.

Beyer, C., J. C. Villar, V. Suwanvanichkij, S. Singh, S. D. Baral, and E. J. Mills. 2007. Health and human rights. 3. Neglected diseases, civil conflicts, and the right to health. *Lancet* **370**:619–627.

Bharti, A. R., J. E. Nally, J. N. Ricaldi, M. A. Matthias, M. M. Diaz, M. A. Lovett, P. N. Levett, R. H. Gilman, M. R. Willig, E. Gotuzzo, J. M. Vinetz, and the Peru-United

States Leptospirosis Consortium. 2003. Leptospirosis: a zoonotic disease of global importance. *Lancet Infect. Dis.* **3:**757–771.

Bisser, S., F. X. N'Siesi, V. Lejon, P. M. Preux, S. Van Nieuwenhove, C. Miaka Mia Bilenge, and P. Büscher. 2007. Equivalence trial of melarsoprol and nifurtimox monotherapy and combination therapy for the treatment of second-stage *Trypanosoma brucei gambiense* sleeping sickness. *J. Infect. Dis.* **195:**322–329.

Blackburn, B. G., A. Eigege, H. Gotau, G. Gerlong, E. Miri, W. A. Hawley, E. Mathieu, and F. Richards. 2006. Successful integration of insecticide-treated bed net distribution with mass drug administration in Central Nigeria. *Am. J. Trop. Med. Hyg.* **75:**650–655.

Bleakley, H. 2006. Disease and development: evidence from hookworm eradication in the American South. Working paper no. 205. George J. Stigler Center for the Study of the Economy and the State, University of Chicago, Chicago, IL. http://research. chicagogsb.edu/economy/research/articles/205.pdf. Accessed 9 February 2008.

Bleakley, H. 2007. Disease and development: evidence from hookworm eradication in the American South. *Q. J. Econ.* **122:**73–112.

Boatin, B. A., and F. O. Richard. 2006. Control of onchocerciasis. *Adv. Parasitol.* **61:** 349–394.

Borkow, G., and Z. Bentwich. 2006. HIV and helminth co-infection. *Parasite Immunol.* **28:**605–612.

Bottazzi, M. E., A. P. Miles, D. Diemert, and P. J. Hotez. 2006. An ounce of prevention on a budget: a nonprofit approach to developing vaccines against neglected diseases. *Expert Rev. Vaccines* **5:**189–198.

Brady, M. A., P. J. Hooper, and E. A. Ottesen. 2006. Projected benefits from integrating NTD programs in sub-Saharan Africa. *Trends Parasitol.* **22:**285–291.

Brentlinger, P. E., L. Capps, and M. Denson. 2003. Hookworm infection and anemia in adult women in rural Chiapas, Mexico. *Salud Publica Mex.* **45:**117–119.

Broder, S., S. L. Hoffman, and P. J. Hotez. 2002. Cures for the Third World's problems: the application of genomics to the diseases plaguing the developing world may have huge medical and economic benefits for those countries and might even prevent armed conflict. *EMBO Rep.* **3:**806–812.

Brooker, S. 2002. Schistosomes, snails and satellites. *Acta Tropica* **82:**207–214.

Brooker, S., W. Akhwale, R. Pullan, B. Estambale, S. E. Clarke, R. W. Snow, and P. J. Hotez. 2007. Epidemiology of plasmodium-helminth co-infection in Africa: populations at risk, potential impact on anemia, and prospects for combining control. *Am. J. Trop. Med. Hyg.* **77:**88–98.

Brooker, S., M. Beasley, M. Ndinaromtan, E. M. Madjiouroum, M. Baboguel, E. Djenguinabe, S. I. Hay, and D. A. Bundy. 2002. Use of remote sending and a geographical information system in a national helminth control programme in Chad. *Bull. W. H. O.* **80:**783–789.

Brooker, S., J. Bethony, and P. J. Hotez. 2004. Human hookworm infection in the 21st century. *Adv. Parasitol.* **58:**197–288.

Brooker, S., A. C. Clements, and D. A. Bundy. 2006a. Global epidemiology, ecology and control of soil-transmitted helminth infections. *Adv. Parasitol.* **62:**221–261.

Brooker, S., A. C. Clements, P. J. Hotez, S. I. Hay, A. J. Tatem, D. A. Bundy, and R. W. Snow. 2006b. The co-distribution of *Plasmodium falciparum* and hookworm among African schoolchildren. *Malar. J.* **5:**99.

Brooker, S., and J. Utzinger. May 2007. Integrated disease mapping in a polyparasitic world. *Geospatial Health* **2:**141–146.

Brownback, S. May 2007, posting date. Brownback applauds adoption of Neglected Diseases Amendment to FDA Revitalization Act. http://brownback.senate.gov/pressapp/record.cfm?id=273870.

Brun, R., and O. Balmer. 2006. New developments in human African trypanosomiasis. *Curr. Opin. Infect. Dis.* **19:**415–430.

Brzezinski, Z. 2004. *The Choice: Global Domination or Global Leadership*, p. 160–217. Basic Books, New York, NY.

Buchan, J. 2006. Visual loss in post-conflict southern Sudan. *PLoS Med.* **3:**e450.

Buijs, J., G. Borsboom, M. Renting, W. J. A. Hilgersom, J. C. van Wieringen, G. Jansen, and J. Neijens. 1997. Relationship between allergic manifestations and Toxocara seropositivity: a cross-sectional study among elementary school children. *Eur. Respir. J.* **10:**1467–1475.

Bundy, D. A., M. S. Chan, and L. Savioli. 1995. Hookworm infection in pregnancy. *Trans. R. Soc. Trop. Med. Hyg.* **89:**521–522.

Burri, C., and R. Brun. 2002. Human African trypanosomiasis, p. 1303–1323. *In* G. C. Cook and A. I. Zumla (ed.), *Manson's Tropical Diseases*, 21st ed. W. B. Saunders, New York, NY.

Busse, W. W., and H. Mitchell. 2007. Addressing issues of asthma in inner-city children. *J. Allerg. Clin. Immunol.* **119:**43–49.

Cachay, E. R., and J. M. Vinetz. 2005. A global research agenda for leptospirosis. *J. Postgrad. Med.* **51:**174–178.

Cairncross, S., R. Muller, and N. Zagaria. 2002. Dracunculiasis (Guinea worm disease) and the eradication initiative. *Clin. Microbiol. Rev.* **15:**223–246.

Campbell, W. C. 1991. Ivermectin as an antiparasitic agent for use in humans. *Annu. Rev. Microbiol.* **45:**445–474.

Canning, D. 2006. Priority setting and the 'neglected' tropical diseases. *Trans. R. Soc. Trop. Med. Hyg.* **100:**499–504.

Capron, A., G. Riveau, M. Capron, and F. Trottein. 2005. Schistosomes: the road from host-parasite interactions to vaccines in clinical trials. *Trends Parasitol.* **21:**143–149.

Carey, H. 1970. A war we can win: health as a vector of foreign policy. Symposium on Medicine and Diplomacy in the Tropics. *Bull. N. Y. Acad. Med.* **46:**334–350.

Carter Center. 2006. *25th Anniversary Annual Report: 2005–2006*, p. 30. Carter Center, Atlanta, GA.

Centers for Disease Control and Prevention. 2002. Cancer death rates—Appalachia, 1994–1998. *Morb. Mortal. Wkly. Rep.* **51**(24):527–529.

Centers for Disease Control and Prevention. 2005. Leptospirosis. Centers for Disease Control and Prevention, Atlanta, GA. http://www.cdc.gov/ncidod/dbmd/diseaseinfo/leptospirosis_t.htm. Accessed 7 February 2008.

Chirac, P., and E. Torreele. 2006. Global framework on essential health R&D. *Lancet* **367:**1560–1561.

Chitsulo, L., D. Engels, A. Montresor, and L. Savioli. 2000. The global status of schistosomiasis and its control. *Acta Tropica* **77:**41–51.

Chorazy, M. L., and D. J. Richardson. 2005. A survey of environmental contamination with ascarid ova, Wallingford, Connecticut. *Vector Borne Zoonotic Dis.* **5:**33–39.

Christian, P., S. K. Khatry, and K. P. West, Jr. 2004. Antenatal anthelmintic treatment, birthweight, and infant survival in rural Nepal. *Lancet* **364:**981–983.

Clancey, J., R. Dodge, and H. F. Lunn. 1962. Study of a mycobacterium causing skin ulceration in Uganda. *Ann. Soc. Belg. Med. Trop.* **42:**585–590.

Cobb, C., Jr. December 2001, posting date. Africa: elimination of river blindness "possible within ten years." http://allafrica.com/stories/200112150001.html.

Coggeshall, L. T. 1945. Malaria and filariasis in the returning serviceman. *Am. J. Trop. Med. Hyg.* **25:**177–196.

Cole, S. T., K. Eiglmeier, J. Parkhill, K. D. James, N. R. Thomson, P. R. Wheeler, N. Honoré, T. Garnier, C. Churcher, D. Harris, K. Mungall, D. Basham, D. Brown, T. Chillingworth, R. Connor, R. M. Davies, K. Devlin, S. Duthoy, T. Feltwell, A. Fraser, N. Hamlin, S. Holroyd, T. Hornsby, K. Jagels, C. Lacroix, J. Maclean, S. Moule, L. Murphy, K. Oliver, M. A. Quail, M. A. Rajandream, K. M. Rutherford, S. Rutter, K. Seeger, S. Simon, M. Simmonds, J. Skelton, R. Squares, S. Squares, K. Stevens, K. Taylor, S. Whitehead, J. R. Woodward, and B. G. Barrell. 2001. Massive gene decay in the leprosy bacillus. *Nature* **409:**1007–1011.

Coleman, P. G., E. M. Fèvre, and S. Cleaveland. 2004. Estimating the public health impact of rabies. *Emerg. Infect. Dis.* **10:**140–142.

Coler, R. N., and S. G. Reed. 2005. Second-generation vaccines against leishmaniasis. *Trends Parasitol.* **21:**244–249.

Collin, S. M., P. G. Coleman, K. Ritmeijer, and R. N. Davidson. 2006. Unseen Kala-azar deaths in south Sudan (1999–2002). *Trop. Med. Int. Health* **11:**509–512.

Conder, G. A., and W. C. Campbell. 1995. Chemotherapy of nematode infections of veterinary importance, with special reference to drug resistance. *Adv. Parasitol.* **35:**1–84.

Conrad, J. 1902. *Heart of Darkness* and *The Secret Sharer*, p. 83. Signet Classics, Penguin Putnam, New York, NY.

Conyer, R. T. 2006. Response from the Mexican Ministry of Health. *Lancet* **368:**1768–1769.

Cotreau, M. M., S. Warren, J. L. Ryan, L. Fleckenstein, S. R. Vanapalli, K. R. Brown, D. Rock, C.-Y. Chen, and U. S. Schwertschlag. 2003. The antiparasitic moxidectin: safety, tolerability, and pharmacokinetics in humans. *J. Clin. Pharmacol.* **43:**1108–1115.

Courtright, P., S. H. Kim, H. S. Lee, and S. Lewallen. 1997. Excess mortality associated with blindness in leprosy patients in Korea. *Lepr. Rev.* **68:**326–330.

Cox, F. E. 2004. History of sleeping sickness (African trypanosomiasis). *Infect. Dis. Clin. N. Am.* **18:**231–245.

Cox, F. E. 2002. History of human parasitology. *Clin. Microbiol. Rev.* **15:**595–612.

Croft, S. L., M. P. Barrett, and J. A. Urbina. 2005. Chemotherapy of trypanosomiases and leishmaniasis. *Trends Parasitol.* **21:**508–512.

Croft, S. L., K. Seifert, and V. Yardley. 2006. Current scenario of drug development for leishmaniasis. *Indian J. Med. Res.* **123:**399–410.

Crompton, D. W. 2000. The public health importance of hookworm disease. *Parasitology* **121**(Suppl.):S39–S50.

Crompton, D. W. 2001. Ascaris and ascariasis. *Adv. Parasitol.* **48:**285–375.

Crompton, D. W., and M. C. Nesheim. 2002. Nutritional impact of intestinal helminthiasis during the human life cycle. *Annu. Rev. Nutr.* **22:**35–59.

Dandona, L., and R. Dandona. 2006. What is the global burden of visual impairment? *BMC Med.* **4:**6.

DeGiorgio, C., S. Pietsch-Escueta, V. Tsang, G. Corral-Leyva, L. Ng, M. T. Medina, S. Astudillo, N. Padilla, P. Levya, L. Martinez, J. Noh, M. Levine, R. del Villasenor, and F. Sorvillo. 2005a. Sero-prevalence of *Taenia solium* cysticercosis and *Taenia solium* taeniasis in California, USA. *Acta Neurol. Scand.* **111:**84–88.

DeGiorgio, C. M., F. Sorvillo, and S. Pietsch-Escueta. 2005b. Neurocysticercosis in the United States: review of an important emerging infection. *Neurology* **64:**1486.

del La Garza, Y., E. A. Graviss, N. G. Daver, K. J. Gambarin, W. X. Shandera, P. M. Schantz, and A. C. White, Jr. 2005. Epidemiology of neurocysticercosis in Houston, Texas. *Am. J. Trop. Med. Hyg.* **73:**766–770.

de Silva, N. R., S. Brooker, P. J. Hotez, A. Montresor, D. Engels, and L. Savioli. 2003. Soil-transmitted helminth infections: updating the global picture. *Trends Parasitol.* **19:**547–551.

Despommier, D. D., R. W. Gwadz, P. J. Hotez, and C. Knirsch. 2006. *Parasitic Diseases*, 5th ed. Apple Tree Productions, New York, NY.

Dickson, R., S. Awasthi, P. Williamson, C. Demellweek, and P. Garner. 2000. Effects of treatment for intestinal helminth infection on growth and cognitive performance in children: systematic review of randomised trials. *BMJ* **320:**1697–1701.

Diemert, D. J., J. M. Bethony, and P. J. Hotez. 2008. Hookworm vaccines. *Clin. Infect. Dis.* **46:**282–288.

Dinh, K. X. 2001. Rabies in humans in Viet Nam, p. 255–256. *In* B. Dodet and F.-X. Meslin (ed.), *Rabies Control in Asia*. John Libbey Eurotext, Paris, France.

Disalvo, A. F., and J. Melonas. 1970. Intestinal parasites in South Carolina, 1969. *J. S. C. Med. Assoc.* **66:**355–358.

Donoghue, H. D., A. Marcsik, C. Matheson, K. Vernon, E. Nuorala, J. E. Molto, C. L. Greenblatt, and M. Spigelman. 2005. Co-infection of *Mycobacterium tuberculosis* and *Mycobacterium leprae* in human archaeological samples: a possible explanation for the historical decline of leprosy. *Proc. Biol. Sci.* **272:**389–394.

Druilhe, P., A. Tall, and C. Sokhna. 2005. Worms can worsen malaria: towards a new means to roll back malaria? *Trends Parasitol.* **21:**359–362.

Dugger, C. W. 2007. U. N. predicts urban population explosion. *N. Y. Times* **2007** (28 June).

Edelman, R. 2007. Dengue vaccines approach the finish line. *Clin. Infect. Dis.* **45**(Suppl. 1):S56–S60.

Ehrenberg, J. P. 2002. *An Epidemiological Overview of Geohelminth and Schistosomiasis in the Caribbean*. Pan American Health Organization, Washington, DC.

El Sayed, N. M., P. J. Myler, G. Blandin, M. Berrlman, et al. 2005. Comparative genomics of trypanosomatid parasitic protozoa. *Science* **309**:404–409.

El-Sayed, N. M., P. J. Myler, D. C. Bartholomeu, et al. 2005. The genome sequence of *Trypanosoma cruzi*, etiologic agent of Chagas disease. *Science* **309**: 409–415.

Enserink, M. 2000. Infectious diseases. Has leishmaniasis become endemic in the U. S.? *Science* **290**:1881–1883.

Erlanger, T. E., J. Keiser, M. C. Castro, R. Bos, B. H. Singer, M. Tanner, and J. Utzinger. 2005. Effect of water resource development and management on lymphatic filariasis, and estimates of populations at risk. *Am. J. Trop. Med. Hyg.* **73**:523–533.

Ettling, J. 1981. *The Germ of Laziness: Rockefeller Philanthropy and Public Health in the New South.* Harvard University Press, Cambridge, MA.

Farley, J. 1991. *Bilharzia: a History of Imperial Tropical Medicine.* Cambridge University Press, Cambridge, United Kingdom.

Farley, J. 2004. *To Cast Out Disease: a History of the International Health Division of the Rockefeller Foundation (1913–1951).* Oxford University Press, Oxford, United Kingdom.

Farmer, H. F. 1983. The germ of laziness: a Florida historical perspective. *J. Fla. Med. Assoc.* **70**:659–662.

Faust, E. C., P. F. Russell, and R. C. Jung. 1970. *Craig and Faust's Clinical Parasitology,* 8th ed., p. 251. Lea & Febiger, Philadelphia, PA.

Fenghua, S., W. Zhongxing, Q. Yixing, C. Hanqun, X. Haichou, R. Hainan, X. Shuhua, Z. Bin, J. M. Hawdon, F. Zheng, and P. J. Hotez. 1998. Epidemiology of human intestinal nematode infections in Wujiang and Pizhou counties, Jiangsu Province, China. *Southeast Asian J. Trop. Med. Public Health* **29**:605–610.

Fenwick, A. 2006. Waterborne infectious diseases—could they be consigned to history? *Science* **313**:1077–1081.

Fenwick, A., D. Molyneux, and V. Nantulya. 2005. Achieving the millennium development goals. *Lancet* **365**:1029–1030.

Fenwick, A., D. Rollinson, and V. Southgate. 2006. Implementation of human schistosomiasis control: challenges and prospects. *Adv. Parasitol.* **61**:567–622.

Fenwick, A., and J. P. Webster. 2006. Schistosomiasis: challenges for control, treatment and drug resistance. *Curr. Opin. Infect. Dis.* **19**:577–582.

Fèvre, E. M., K. Picozzi, J. Jannin, S. C. Welburn, and I. Maudlin. 2006. Human African trypanosomiasis: epidemiology and control. *Adv. Parasitol.* **61**:168–221.

Fiftieth World Health Assembly. 1997a. Agenda item 20. Eradication of dracunculiasis. Fiftieth World Health Assembly. http://www.who.int/dracunculiasis/eradication/WHA50.35.pdf. Accessed 11 February 2008.

Fiftieth World Health Assembly. 1997b. Elimination of lymphatic filariasis as a public health problem. Fiftieth World Health Assembly. http://www.who.int/lymphatic_filariasis/resources/WHA_50%2029.pdf.

Fleming, A. F. 1994. Agriculture-related anemias. *Br. J. Biomed. Sci.* **31**:345–357.

Fleming, F. M., S. Brooker, S. M. Geiger, I. R. Caldas, R. Correa-Oliveira, P. J. Hotez, and J. M. Bethony. 2006. Synergistic associations between hookworm and other helminth species in a rural community in Brazil. *Trop. Med. Int. Health* **11**:56–64.

Flisser, A., A. Velasco-Villa, C. Martinez-Campos, F. Gonzalez-Dominguez, B. Briseno-Garcia, R. Garcia-Suarez, A. Caballero-Servin, I. Hernandez-Monroy, H. Garcia-Lozano, L. Gutierrez-Cogco, G. Rodriguez-Angeles, I. Lopez-Martinez, S. Galindo-Virgen, R. Vazquez-Campuzano, S. Balandrano-Campos, C. Guzman-Bracho, A. Olivo-Diaz, J. de la Rosa, C. Magos, A. Escobar-Gutierrez, and D. Correa. 2002. Infectious diseases in Mexico: a survey from 1995–2000. *Arch. Med. Res.* **33:**343–350.

Frick, K. D., E. V. Basilion, C. L. Hanson, and M. A. Colchero. 2003a. Estimating the burden and economic impact of trachomatous visual loss. *Ophthalmic Epidemiol.* **10:**121–132.

Frick, K. D., C. L. Hanson, and G. A. Jacobson. 2003b. Global burden of trachoma and economics of the disease. *Am. J. Trop. Med. Hyg.* **69**(Suppl. 5):1–10.

Furman, B. 1973. *A Profile of the United States Public Health Service 1798–1948*, p. 308–311. Publication no. (NIH) 73-369. U.S. Department of Health, Education and Welfare, U. S. Government Printing Office, Washington, DC. http://fortyandeight.org/thestar/carville/carville_history.htm. Accessed 9 February 2008.

Gallagher, M., I. Malhotra, P. L. Mungai, A. N. Wamachi, J. M. Kioko, J. H. Ouma, E. Muchiri, and C. L. King. 2005. The effects of maternal helminth and malaria infections on mother-to-child HIV transmission. *AIDS* **19:**1849–1855.

Gallup, J. L., and J. D. Sachs. 2001. The economic burden of malaria. *Am. J. Trop. Med. Hyg.* **64**(Suppl. 1–2):85–96.

Gaudet, M. 2004. *Carville: Remembering Leprosy in America*. University Press of Mississippi, Jackson.

Geary, T. G. 2005. Ivermectin 20 years on: maturation of a wonder drug. *Trends Parasitol.* **21:**530–532.

George, K. M., D. Chatterjee, G. Gunawardana, D. Welty, J. Hayman, R. Lee, and P. L. Small. 1999. Mycolactone: a polyketide toxin from *Mycobacterium ulcerans* required for virulence. *Science* **283:**854–857.

Global Alliance to Eliminate Lymphatic Filariasis. 2004. The socio-economic impact of LF and the program to eliminate it. Task Force for Child Survival and Development, Lymphatic Filariasis Support Center, Decatur, GA. http://www.taskforce.org/lfsc/toolkit/overview/SEBurden.pdf. Accessed 9 February 2008.

Goozner, M. 2007. Stopping hookworm. *Scientist* **2007**(July): 52–59.

Greenwood, B. 2006. Review: intermittent preventive treatment—a new approach to the prevention of malaria in children in areas with seasonal malaria transmission. *Trop. Med. Int. Health* **11:**983–991.

Greenwood, K., T. Williams, and T. Geary. 2005. Nematode neuropeptide receptors and their development as anthelmintic screens. *Parasitology* **131**(Suppl.):S169–S177.

Grove, D. I. 1990. *A History of Human Helminthology*. CAB International, Wallingford, United Kingdom.

Gryseels, B., K. Polman, J. Clerinx, and L. Kestens. 2006. Human schistosomiasis. *Lancet* **368:**1106–1118.

Gubler, D. J., and G. G. Clark. 1995. Dengue/dengue hemorrhagic fever: the emergence of a global health problem. *Emerg. Infect. Dis.* **1:**55–57.

Gubler, D. J., P. Reiter, K. L. Ebi, W. Yap, R. Nasci, and J. A. Patz. 2001. Climate variability and change in the United States: potential impacts on vector- and rodent-borne diseases. *Environ. Health Perspect.* **109**(Suppl. 2):223–233.

Guha-Sapir, D., and W. G. van Panhuis. 2002. Armed conflict and public health: a report on knowledge and knowledge gaps. WHO Collaborating Center for Research on the Epidemiology of Disasters, Brussels, Belgium. http://www.cred.be/docs/cred/publications/rocpressweb.pdf. Accessed 9 February 2008.

Guyatt, H. L., and R. W. Snow. 2004. Impact of malaria during pregnancy on low birth weight in sub-Saharan Africa. *Clin. Microbiol. Rev.* **17**:760–769.

Guzik, D. 2004. Leviticus 13: the diagnosis of leprosy. Enduring Word Media, Ventura, CA. http://www.enduringword.com/commentaries/0313.htm. Accessed 9 February 2008.

Halstead, S. B. 1981. The pathogenesis of dengue: the Alexander D. Langmuir Lecture. *Am. J. Trop. Med. Hyg.* **114**:632–648.

Hanford, E. T., B. F. Zhan, Y. Lu, and A. Giordano. 2007. Chagas disease in Texas: recognizing the significance and implications of evidence in the literature. *Soc. Sci. Med.* **65**:60–79.

Harrison, G. A. 1978. *Mosquitoes, Malaria, and Man: a History of the Hostilities since 1880*, p. 242–254. E. P. Dutton, New York, NY.

Hathaway, W. 2007. Whole new level of care. *Hartford Courant* **2007**(13 May).

Hawking, F. 1955. The chemotherapy of filarial infections. *Pharmacol. Rev.* **7**:279–299.

Hawking, F. 1958. Filariasis. *Sci. Am.* **199**:94–101.

Hawking, F., and R. J. Marques. 1967. Control of bancroftian filariasis by cooking salt medicated with diethylcarbamazine. *Bull. W. H. O.* **37**:405–414.

Hawking, F., P. Sewell, and J. P. Thurston. 1950. The mode of action of hetrazan on filarial worms. *Br. J. Pharmacol.* **5**:217–238.

Haynes, D. M. 2001. *Imperial Medicine: Patrick Manson and the Conquest of Tropical Disease.* University of Pennsylvania Press, Philadelphia.

Healy, G. R., N. N. Gleason, R. Bokat, H. Pond, and M. Roper. 1969. Prevalence of ascariasis and amebiasis in Cherokee Indian school children. *Public Health Rep.* **84**:907–914.

Henderson, H. E. 1957. Incidence and intensity of hookworm infestation in certain East Texas counties with comparison of technics. *Tex. Rep. Biol. Med.* **15**:283–292.

Hermann, N., L. T. Glickman, P. M. Schantz, M. G. Weston, and L. M. Domanski. 1985. Seroprevalence of zoonotic toxocariasis in the United States: 1971–1973. *Am. J. Epidemiol.* **122**:890–896.

Heukelbach, J., F. A. de Oliveira, L. R. Kerr-Pontes, and H. Feldmeier. 2001. Risk factors associated with an outbreak of dengue fever in a favela in Fortaleza, north-east Brazil. *Trop. Med. Int. Health* **6**:635–642.

Hillyer, G. V. 2005. The rise and fall of Bilharzia in Puerto Rico: its centennial 1904–2004. *P. R. Health Sci. J.* **24**:225–235.

Hlvasa, M. C., J. C. Watson, and M. J. Beach. 2005. Giardiasis surveillance—United States, 1998–2002. *Morb. Mortal. Wkly. Rep. Surveill. Summ.* **54**:9–16.

Holland, C. V., D. L. Taren, D. W. Crompton, M. C. Nesheim, D. Sanjur, I. Barbeau, K. Tucker, J. Tiffany, and G. Rivera. 1988. Intestinal helminthiases in relation to the socioeconomic environment of Panamanian children. *Soc. Sci. Med.* **26:**209–213.

Hopkins, D. R., E. Ruiz-Tiben, P. Downs, P. C. Withers, Jr., and J. H. Maguire. 2005. Dracunculiasis eradication: the final inch. *Am. J. Trop. Med. Hyg.* **73:**669–675.

Hopkins, D. R., and P. C. Withers, Jr. 2002. Sudan's war and eradication of dracunculiasis. *Lancet* **360**(Suppl.):s21–s22.

Hoppe, K. A. 2003. *Lords of the Fly: Sleeping Sickness Control in British East Africa, 1900–1960.* Praeger, Westport, CT.

Horn, J. S. 1969. *Away with All Pests: an English Surgeon in People's China, 1954–1969*, p. 94–106. Monthly Review Press, New York, NY.

Horton, J. 2003. Global anthelmintic chemotherapy programs: learning from history. *Trends Parasitol.* **19:**405–409.

Hotez, P. 2002a. Appeasing Wilson's ghost: the expanded role of the new vaccines in international foreign policy. Health and Security Series occasional paper no. 3. Chemical and Biological Arms Control Institute, Washington, DC.

Hotez, P., E. Ottesen, A. Fenwick, and D. Molyneux. 2006a. The neglected tropical diseases: the ancient afflictions of stigma and poverty and the prospects for their control and elimination. *Adv. Exp. Biol. Med.* **582:**23–33.

Hotez, P., S. Raff, A. Fenwick, F. Richards, Jr., and D. H. Molyneux. 2007a. Recent progress in integrated neglected tropical disease control. *Trends Parasitol.* **23:**511–514.

Hotez, P. J. 2001a. Vaccine diplomacy. *Foreign Policy* **2001**(May–June):68–69.

Hotez, P. J. 2001b. Vaccines as instruments of foreign policy. *EMBO Rep.* **2:**862–868.

Hotez, P. J. 2002b. China's hookworms. *China Q.* **172:**1029–1041.

Hotez, P. J. 2002c. Reducing the global burden of human parasitic diseases. *Comp. Parasitol.* **69:**140–145.

Hotez, P. J. 2004. The National Institutes of Health roadmap and the developing world. *J. Investig. Med.* **52:**246–247.

Hotez, P. J. 2006. The "biblical diseases" and U. S. vaccine diplomacy. *Brown J. W. Aff.* **12**(2):247–258.

Hotez, P. J. 2007a. Hookworm and poverty. *Ann. N. Y. Acad. Sci.* Epub ahead of print.

Hotez, P. J. 2007b. Control of onchocerciasis—the next generation. *Lancet* **369:**1979–1980.

Hotez, P. J., J. Bethony, M. E. Bottazzi, S. Brooker, and P. Buss. 2005. Hookworm: "the great infection of mankind." *PLoS Med.* **2:**e67.

Hotez, P. J., J. Bethony, M. E. Bottazzi, S. Brooker, D. Diemert, and A. Loukas. 2006b. New technologies for the control of human hookworm infection. *Trends Parasitol.* **22:**327–331.

Hotez, P. J., S. Brooker, J. M. Bethony, M. E. Bottazzi, A. Loukas, and S. H. Xiao. 2004. Hookworm infection. *N. Engl. J. Med.* **351:**799–807.

Hotez, P. J., D. A. P. Bundy, K. Beegle, S. Brooker, L. Drake, N. de Silva, A. Montresor, D. Engels, M. Jukes, L. Chitsulo, J. Chow, R. Laxminarayan, C. M. Michaud, J. Bethony, R. Correa-Oliveira, S. H. Xiao, A. Fenwick, and L. Savioli. 2006c. Helminth infections: soil-transmitted helminth infections and schistosomiasis, p. 467–482. *In* D. T. Jamison, J. G. Breman, A. R. Measham, G. Alleyne, M. Claeson, D. B. Evans, J. Prabhat, A. Mills, and P. Musgrove (ed.), *Disease Control Priorities in Developing Countries*, 2nd ed. Oxford University Press, Oxford, United Kingdom.

Hotez, P. J., and M. T. Ferris. 2006. The antipoverty vaccines. *Vaccine* **24:**5787–5799.

Hotez, P. J., D. H. Molyneux, A. Fenwick, J. Kumaresan, S. Ehrlich, Sachs, J. D. Sachs, and L. Savioli. 2007b. Control of neglected tropical diseases. *N. Engl. J. Med.* **357:**1018–1027.

Hotez, P. J., D. H. Molyneux, A. Fenwick, E. Ottesen, S. Ehrlich Sachs, and J. D. Sachs. 2006d. Incorporating a rapid-impact package for neglected tropical diseases with programs for HIV/AIDS, tuberculosis, and malaria. *PLoS Med.* **3:**e102.

Hotez, P. J., E. Ottesen, A. Fenwick, and D. Molyneux. 2006e. The neglected tropical diseases: the ancient afflictions of stigma and poverty and the prospects for their control and elimination. *Adv. Exp. Med. Biol.* **582:**23–33.

Hotez, P. J., F. Zheng, X. Long-qi, C. Ming-gang, X. Shu-hua, L. Shi-xian, D. Blair, D. P. McManus, and G. M. Davis. 1997. Emerging and reemerging helminthiases and the public health of China. *Emerg. Infect. Dis.* **3:**303–310.

Houston, R. 2000. Salt fortified with diethylcarbamazine (DEC) as an effective intervention for lymphatic filariasis, with lessons learned from salt iodization programs. *Parasitology* **121:**S161–S173.

Hulse, E. V. 1971. Joshua's curse and the abandonment of ancient Jericho: schistosomiasis as a possible medical explanation. *Med. Hist.* **15:**376–386.

Humphreys, M. 2001. *Malaria, Poverty, Race, and Public Health in the United States,* p. 110–111. The Johns Hopkins University Press, Baltimore, MD.

Hunt, P. 2006. The human right to the highest attainable standard of health: new opportunities and challenges. *Trans. R. Soc. Trop. Med. Hyg.* **100:**603–607.

Ichimori, K., P. M. Graves, and A. Crump. 2007. Lymphatic filariasis elimination in the Pacific: PacELF replicating Japanese success. *Trends Parasitol.* **23:**36–40.

Institute for One World Health. 2008. Visceral leishmaniasis. Institute for One World Health, San Francisco, CA. http://www.oneworldhealth.org/diseases/leishmaniasis.php?PHPSESSID=8818cf0696a7a50ef6d7f8c022d5a9f0. Accessed 11 February 2008.

International Bank for Reconstruction and Development. 2004. Pages from World Bank history: the fight against riverblindness. The World Bank Group, Washington, DC. http://go.worldbank.org/CO9LM3GDZ0. Accessed 9 February 2008.

International Trachoma Initiative. 2006. The Kingdom of Morocco. International Trachoma Initiative, New York, NY. http://www.trachoma.org/cpropdf/Morocco.pdf. Accessed 9 February 2008.

International Trachoma Initiative. 2008. Zithromax® in the control of blinding trachoma: a program manager's guide. International Trachoma Initiative, New York, NY. www.trachoma.org

Jacobson, S. 2007. Rare, non-fatal skin disease found in N. Texans. *Dallas Morning News* **2007**(14 September).

John, T. J. 2005. The prevention and control of human leptospirosis. *J. Postgrad. Med.* **51:**205–209.

Johnson, P. D. R., T. Stinear, P. L. C. Small, G. Plushke, R. W. Merritt, F. Portaels, K. Huygen, J. A. Hayman, and K. Asiedu. 2005. Buruli ulcer (*M. ulcerans* infection): new insights, new hope for disease control. *PLoS Med.* **2:**e108.

Jones, J. L., D. Kruszon-Moran, and M. Wilson. 2003. *Toxoplasma gondii* infection in the United States, 1999–2000. *Emerg. Infect. Dis.* **9:**1371–1374.

Kabatereine, N. B., F. M. Fleming, U. Nyandindi, J. C. Mwanza, and L. Blair. 2006. The control of schistosomiasis and soil-transmitted helminths in East Africa. *Trends Parasitol.* **22:**332–339.

Kale, O. O. 1998. Onchocerciasis: the burden of disease. *Ann. Trop. Med. Parasitol.* **92**(Suppl. 1):S101–S115.

Kaminsky, R., P. Ducray, M. Jung, R. Clover, L. Rufener, J. Bouvier, S. S. Weber, A. Wenger, S. Wieland-Burghausen, T. Goebel, N. Gauvry, F. Pautrat, T. Skirpsky, O. Froelich, C. Komoin-Oka, B. Westlund, A. Sluder, and P. Mäser. 2008. A new class of anthelmintics effective against drug-resistant nematodes. *Nature* **452:**176–180.

Kasi, P. M., A. I. Gilani, K. Ahmad, and N. Z. Janjua. 2004. Blinding trachoma: a disease of poverty. *PLoS Med.* **1:**e44.

Kay, B. H., V. S. Nam, T. V. Tien, N. T. Yen, T. V. Phong, V. T. Diep, T. U. Ninh, A. Bektas, and J. G. Aaskov. 2002. Control of Aedes vectors of dengue in three provinces of Vietnam by use of Mesocyclops (Copepoda) and community-based methods validated by entomologic, clinical, and serological surveillance. *Am. J. Trop. Med. Hyg.* **66:**40–48.

Kennedy, P. G. 2006. Human African trypanosomiasis—neurological aspects. *J. Neurol.* **253:**411–416.

Kernan, F. A. J. 1959. The blood fluke that saved Formosa. *Harper's Magazine* **1959**(April):45–47.

Kessel, J. F., G. C. Thooris, and B. Bambridge. 1953. The use of diethylcarbamazine (hetrazan or notezine) in Tahiti as an aid in the control of filariasis. *Am. J. Trop. Med. Hyg.* **2:**1050–1061.

Kim, A., A. Tandon, and E. Ruiz-Tiben. 1997. Cost-benefit analysis of the global dracunculiasis eradication campaign. Policy research working paper 1835. Africa Human Development Department, World Bank, Washington, DC.

Kim, K. 2006. Time to screen for congenital toxoplasmosis? *Clin. Infect. Dis.* **42:**1395–1397.

King, C. H. 2007. Lifting the burden of schistosomiasis—defining elements of infection-associated disease and the benefits of antiparasite treatment. *J. Infect. Dis.* **196:**653–655.

King, C. H., K. Dickman, and D. J. Tisch. 2005. Reassessment of the cost of chronic helmintic infection: a meta-analysis of disability-related outcomes in endemic schistosomiasis. *Lancet* **365:**1561–1569.

King, C. H., R. F. Sturrock, H. C. Kariuki, and J. Hamburger. 2006. Transmission control for schistosomiasis—why it matters now. *Trends Parasitol.* **22:**575–582.

Kishore, S. P., and P. S. Dhadialla. 2007. A student-led campaign to help tackle neglected tropical diseases. *PLoS Med.* **4:**e241.

Kissinger, H. 2001. *Does America Need a Foreign Policy? Toward a Diplomacy for the 21st Century*, p. 18–27. Simon & Schuster, New York, NY.

Kjetland, E. F., P. D. Ndhlovu, E. Gomo, T. Mduluza, N. Midzi, L. Gwanzura, P. R. Mason, L. Sandvik, H. Friis, and S. G. Gundersen. 2006. Association between genital schistosomiasis and HIV in rural Zimbabwean women. *AIDS* **20:**593–600.

Klintowitz, J. 1989. *A Arte do Comércio II — São Paulo 1930–1954.* SENAC, São Paulo, Brazil.

Knipe, D. M., and P. M. Hawley (ed.). 2007. *Fields Virology,* 5th ed. Lippincott Williams & Wilkins, Philadelphia, PA.

Koberle, F. 1968. Chagas' disease and Chagas' disease syndrome: the pathology of American trypanosomiasis. *Adv. Parasitol.* **6:**63–116.

Kremer, M., and R. Glennerster. 2004. *Strong Medicine: Creating Incentives for Pharmaceutical Research on Neglected Diseases.* Princeton University Press, Princeton, NJ.

Kristof, N. 2007. Attack of the worms. *N. Y. Times* **2007**(2 July).

Kroeger, A., M. Nathan, J. Hombach, and the World Health Organization TDR Reference Group on Dengue. 2004. Dengue. *Nat. Rev. Microbiol.* **2:**360–361.

Kuk, S., E. Ozel, H. Oguzturk, G. Kirkil, and M. Kaplan. 2006. Seroprevalence of Toxocara antibodies in patients with adult asthma. *South. Med. J.* **99:**719–722.

Kumaresan, J. 2005. Can blinding trachoma be eliminated by 2020? *Eye* **19:**1067–1073.

Lammie, P. J., A. Fenwick, and J. Utzinger. 2006. A blueprint for success: integration of neglected tropical disease control programmes. *Trends Parasitol.* **22:**313–321.

Lammie, P. J., J. F. Lindo, W. E. Secor, J. Vasquez, S. K. Ault, and M. L. Eberhard. 2007. Eliminating lymphatic filariasis, onchocerciasis and schistosomiasis from the Americas: breaking a historical legacy of slavery. *PLoS Negl. Trop. Dis.* **1:**e71.

Lampton, D. M. 1974. Health policy during the Great Leap Forward. *China Q.* **60:**668–698.

Laxminarayan, R., A. J. Mills, J. G. Breman, A. R. Measham, G. Alleyne, M. Claeson, P. Jha, P. Musgrove, J. Chow, S. Shahid-Salles, and D. T. Jamison. 2006. Advancement of global health: key messages from the Disease Control Priorities Project. *Lancet* **367:**1193–1208.

Lazowski, P. 2004. *Understanding Your Neighbor's Faith: What Christians and Jews Should Know about Each Other.* KTAV Publishing House, Jersey City, NJ.

Leprosy Group, WHO. 2002. Leprosy, p. 1065–1084. *In* G. C. Cook and A. I. Zumla (ed.), *Manson's Tropical Diseases,* 21st ed. W. B. Saunders, New York, NY.

Lerner, B. H. 2005. Remembering Berton Roueché—master of medical mysteries. *N. Engl. J. Med.* **353:**2428–2431.

Levine, R., et al. 2004. *Millions Saved: Proven Successes in Global Health.* Center for Global Development, Washington, DC.

Lewinsohn, R. 2003. Prophet in his own country: Carlos Chagas and the Nobel Prize. *Perspect. Biol. Med.* **46:**532–549.

Lockwood, D. N. J. 2004. Leprosy and poverty. *Int. J. Epidemiol.* **33:**269–270.

Lockwood, D. N. J., and A. Suneetha. 2005. Leprosy: too complex a disease for a simple elimination paradigm. *Bull. W. H. O.* **83:**230–235.

Lopez, A., V. J. Dietz, M. Wilson, T. R. Navin, and J. L. Jones. 2000. Preventing congenital toxoplasmosis. *Morb. Mortal. Wkly. Rep.* **49**(RR02):57–75.

Lubega, G. W., D. K. Byarugaba, and R. K. Prichard. 2002. Immunization with a tubulin-rich preparation from *Trypanosoma brucei* confers broad protection against African trypanosomiasis. *Exp. Parasitol.* **102:**9–22.

Ludlam, J. A. 1978. Prevalence of trachoma among Navajo Indian children. *Am. J. Optom. Physiol. Opt.* **55:**116–118.

Mabaso, M. L. H., C. C. Appleton, J. C. Hughes, and E. Gouws. 2004. Hookworm (*Necator americanus*) transmission in inland areas of sandy soils in KwaZulu-Natal, South Africa. *Trop. Med. Int. Health* **9:**471–476.

Mabaso, M. L. H., C. C. Appleton, J. C. Hughes, and E. Gouws. 2003. The effect of soil type and climate on hookworm (*Necator americanus*) distribution in KwaZulu-Natal, South Africa. *Trop. Med. Int. Health* **8:**722–727.

MacLean, J. D., L. Poirier, T. W. Gyorkos, J. F. Proulx, J. Bourgeault, A. Corriveau, S. Illistiuk, and M. Staudt. 1992. Epidemiologic and serologic definition of primary and secondary trichinosis in the Arctic. *J. Infect. Dis.* **165:**908–912.

MacLean, J. D., J. Viallet, C. Law, and M. Staudt. 1989. Trichinosis in the Canadian Arctic: report of five outbreaks and a new clinical syndrome. *J. Infect. Dis.* **160:**513–520.

Mahoney, R. T., A. Krattiger, J. D. Clemens, and R. Curtiss III. 2007. The introduction of new vaccines into developing countries. IV. Global access strategies. *Vaccine* **25:**4003–4011.

Mahoney, R. T., and J. E. Maynard. 1999. The introduction of new vaccines into developing countries. *Vaccine* **17:**646–652.

Malavige, G. N., S. Fernando, D. J. Fernando, and S. L. Seneviratne. 2004. Dengue viral infections. *Postgrad. Med. J.* **80:**588–601.

Maloney, D. M., J. E. Maloney, D. Dotson, V. L. Popov, and R. L. Sanchez. 2002. Cutaneous leishmaniasis: Texas case diagnosed by electron microscopy. *J. Am. Acad. Dermatol.* **47:**614–616.

Marin-Neto, J. A., E. Cunha-Neto, B. C. Maciel, and M. V. Simões. 2007. Pathogenesis of chronic Chagas heart disease. *Circulation* **115:**1109–1123.

Marmor, M., L. Glickman, F. Shofer, L. A. Faich, C. Rosenberg, B. Cornblatt, and S. Friedman. 1987. Toxocara canis infection of children: epidemiologic and neuropsychologic findings. *Am. J. Public Health* **77:**554–559.

Martin, L. K. 1972. Hookworm in Georgia. I. Survey of intestinal helminth infections and anemia in rural school children. *Am. J. Trop. Med. Hyg.* **31:**919–929.

Martin, M. G., and M. E. Humphreys. 2006. Social consequences of disease in the American South, 1900–World War II. *South. Med. J.* **99:**862–864.

Mathis, A. M., J. L. Holman, L. M. Sturk, M. A. Ismail, D. W. Boykin, R. R. Tidwell, and J. E. Hall. 2006. Accumulation and intracellular distribution of antitrypanosomal diamidine compounds DB75 and DB820 in African trypanosomes. *Antimicrob. Agents Chemother.* **50:**2185–2191.

McBride, A. J., D. A. Athanazio, M. G. Reis, and A. L. Ko. 2005. Leptospirosis. *Curr. Opin. Infect. Dis.* **18:**376–386.

McDonald, J. C., T. W. Gyorkos, B. Alberton, J. D. MacLean, G. Richer, and D. Juranek. 1990. An outbreak of toxoplasmosis in pregnant women in northern Quebec. *J. Infect. Dis.* **161:**769–774.

McGavin, D. D. M. 2002. Ophthalmology in the tropics and subtropics, p. 301. *In* G. C. Cook and A. I. Zumla (ed.), *Manson's Tropical Diseases*, 21st ed. W. B. Saunders, New York, NY.

McKenzie, F. E. 2005. Polyparasitism. *Int. J. Parasitol.* **34:**221–222.

McKerrow, J. H. 2005. Designing drugs for parasitic diseases of the developing world. *PLoS Med.* **2:**e210.

McLeod, R., K. Boyer, T. Karrison, K. Kasza, C. Swisher, N. Roizen, J. Jalbrzikowski, J. Remington, P. Heydemann, A. G. Noble, M. Mets, E. Holfels, S. Withers, P. Latkany, P. Meier, and the Toxoplasmosis Study Group. 2006. Outcome of treatment for congenital toxoplasmosis, 1981–2004: the National Collaborative Chicago-Based, Congenital Toxoplasmosis Study. *Clin. Infect. Dis.* **42:**1383–1394.

McNeil, D. G. Jr. 2006. Dose of tenacity wears down an ancient horror. *N. Y. Times* **2006**(26 March).

Meltzer, M. I., and C. E. Rupprecht. 1998. A review of the economics of the prevention and control of rabies. Part 1. Global impact and rabies in humans. *Pharmacoeconomics* **14:**365–383.

Michael, E., D. A. Bundy, and B. T. Grenfell. 1996. Re-assessing the global prevalence and distribution of lymphatic filariasis. *Parasitology* **112:**409–428.

Miguel, E. A., and M. Kremer. 2003. Worms: identifying impacts on education and health in the presence of treatment externalities. *Econometrica* **72:**159–217.

Miles, M. A. 2002. American trypanosomiasis (Chagas disease), p. 1325–1338. *In* G. C. Cook and A. I. Zumla (ed.), *Manson's Tropical Diseases*, 21st ed. W. B. Saunders, New York, NY.

Molyneux, D. H., P. J. Hotez, and A. Fenwick. 2005. "Rapid-impact interventions": how a policy of integrated control for Africa's neglected tropical diseases could benefit the poor. *PLoS Med.* **2:**e336.

Moran, M. 2005. A breakthrough in R&D for neglected diseases: new ways to get the drugs we need. *PLoS Med.* **2:**e302.

Morel, C. M., T. Acharya, D. Broun, A. Dangi, C. Elias, N. K. Ganguly, C. A. Gardner, R. K. Gupta, J. Haycock, A. D. Heher, P. J. Hotez, H. E. Kettler, G. T. Keusch, A. F. Krattiger, F. T. Kreutz, S. Lall, K. Lee, R. Mahoney, A. Martinez-Palomo, R. A. Mashelkar, S. A. Matlin, M. Mzimba, J. Oehler, R. G. Ridley, P. Senanayake, P. Singer, and M. Yun. 2005. Health innovation networks to help developing countries address neglected diseases. *Science* **309:**401–404.

Murray, H. W., J. D. Berman, C. R. Davies, and N. G. Saravia. 2005. Advances in leishmaniasis. *Lancet* **366:**1561–1577.

Nair, D. 2001. Screening for Strongyloides infection among the institutionalized mentally disabled. *J. Am. Board Fam. Pract.* **14:**51–53.

Naval and Overseas Health Association. 2001–2008. Human African trypanosomiasis (sleeping sickness). Naval and Overseas Health Association, Paris, France. http://www.asnom.org/en/441_trypanosomiase.html. Accessed 9 February 2008.

Ngondi, J., F. Ole-Sempele, A. Onsarigo, I. Matende, S. Baba, M. Reacher, F. Matthews, C. Brayne, and P. M. Emerson. 2006. Prevalence and causes of blindness and low vision in southern Sudan. *PLoS Med.* **3:**e477.

Nimmannitya, S. 2002. Dengue and dengue haemorrhagic fever, p. 765–772. *In* G. C. Cook and A. I. Zumla (ed.), *Manson's Tropical Diseases*, 21st ed. W. B. Saunders, New York, NY.

Nokes, C., S. M. Grantham-McGregor, A. W. Sawyer, E. S. Cooper, and D. A. Bundy. 1992. Parasitic helminth infection and cognitive function in school children. *Proc. Biol. Sci.* **247:**77–81.

Ntab, B., B. Cisse, D. Boulanger, C. Sokhna, G. Targett, J. Lines, N. Alexander, J. F. Trape, F. Simondon, B. M. Greenwood, and K. B. Simondon. 2007. Impact of intermittent preventive anti-malarial treatment on the growth and nutritional status of preschool children in rural Senegal (West Africa). *Am. J. Trop. Med. Hyg.* **77:**411–417.

Nutman, T. B., and V. Kumaraswami. 2001. Regulation of the immune response in lymphatic filariasis: perspectives on acute and chronic infection with *Wuchereria bancrofti* in South India. *Parasite Immunol.* **23:**389–399.

Nye, J. S., Jr. 1999. Redefining the national interest. *Foreign Aff.* **1999**(July/August).

Odiit, M., A. Shaw, S. C. Welburn, E. M. Fèvre, P. G. Coleman, and J. J. McDermott. 2004. Assessing the patterns of health-seeking behaviour and awareness among sleeping-sickness patients in eastern Uganda. *Ann. Trop. Med. Parasitol.* **98:**329–348.

Ong, S., D. A. Talan, G. J. Moran, W. Mower, M. Newdow, V. C. Tsang, R. W. Pinner, and the EMERGEncy ID NET Study Group. 2002. Neurocysticercosis in radiographically imaged seizure patients in U. S. emergency departments. *Emerg. Infect. Dis.* **8:**608–613.

Osei-Atweneboana, M. Y., J. K. Eng, D. A. Boakye, J. O. Gyapoing, and R. K. Prichard. 2007. Prevalence and intensity of *Onchocerca volvulus* infection and efficacy of ivermectin in endemic communities in Ghana: a two-phase epidemiological study. *Lancet* **369:**2021–2029.

Ottesen, E. A. 2006. Lymphatic filariasis: treatment, control and elimination. *Adv. Parasitol.* **61:**395–441.

Pan American Health Organization. 2007. 2006: number of reported cases of dengue & dengue hemorrhagic fever (DHF), region of the Americas (by country and subregion). Pan American Health Organization, Washington, DC. http://www.paho.org/english/ad/dpc/cd/dengue-cases-2006.htm. Accessed 9 February 2008.

Pays, E., L. Vanhamme, and D. Perez-Morga. 2004. Antigenic variation in Trypanosoma brucei: facts, challenges, and mysteries. *Curr. Opin. Microbiol.* **7:**369–374.

Pays, E., B. Vanhollebeke, L. Vanhamme, F. Paturiaux-Hanocq, D. P. Nolan, and D. Pérez-Morga. 2006. The trypanolytic factor of human serum. *Nat. Rev. Microbiol.* **4:**477–486.

Pearce, L. 1921. Studies on the treatment of human trypanosomiasis with tryparsamide (the sodium salt of N-phenylglycineamide-p-arsonic acid). *J. Exp. Med.* **24:**1–104.

Pecoul, B. 2004. New drugs for neglected diseases: from pipeline to patients. *PLoS Med.* **1:**e13.

Pepin, J. 2007. Combination therapy for sleeping sickness: a wake-up call. *J. Infect. Dis.* **195:**311–313.

Pepin, J. J., and H. A. Meda. 2001. The epidemiology and control of human African trypanosomiasis. *Adv. Parasitol.* **49:**71–132.

Perera, M., M. Whitehead, D. Molyneux, M. Weerasooriya, and G. Gunatilleke. 2007. Neglected patients with a neglected disease? A qualitative study of lymphatic filariasis. *PLoS Negl. Trop. Dis.* **21:**e128.

Pew Forum on Religion & Public Life. 2002. Religion on the stump: politics and faith in America. Pew Forum on Religion & Public Life, Washington, DC. http://pewforum. org/events/?EventID=34. Accessed 9 February 2008.

Plorde, J. J. 2004. Mycobacteria, p. 439–456. *In* K. J. Ryan and C. G. Ray (ed.), *Sherris Medical Microbiology*, 4th ed. McGraw-Hill Medical Publishing Division, New York, NY.

Portaels, F., P. Eisen, A. Cuimaraes-Peres, P. A. Fonteyne, and W. M. Meyers. 1999. Insects in the transmission of *Mycobacterium ulcerans* infection. *Lancet* **353:**986.

Power, H. J. 1999. *Tropical Medicine in the Twentieth Century: a History of the Liverpool School of Tropical Medicine 1898–1990.* Kegan Paul International, London, United Kingdom.

Prichard, R. K. 2007. Markers for benzimidazole resistance in human parasitic nematodes? *Parasitology* **134:**1987–1992.

Proulx, J.-F., J. D. MacLean, T. W. Gyorkos, D. Leclair, A.-K. Richter, B. Serhir, L. Forbes, and A. A. Gajadhr. 2002. Novel prevention program for trichinellosis in Inuit communities. *Clin. Infect. Dis.* **34:**1508–1514.

Quihui-Cota, L., M. E. Valencia, D. W. Crompton, S. Phillips, P. Hagan, S. P. Diaz-Camacho, and A. Triana-Tejas. 2004. Prevalence and intensity of intestinal parasitic infections in relation to nutritional status in Mexican schoolchildren. *Trans. R. Soc. Trop. Med. Hyg.* **98:**653–659.

Rajan, T. V. 2005. Natural course of lymphatic filariasis: insights from epidemiology, experimental human infections, and clinical observations. *Am. J. Trop. Med. Hyg.* **73:**995–998.

Ramaiah, K. D., P. K. Das, E. Michael, and H. Guyatt. 2000a. The economic burden of lymphatic filariasis. *Parasitol. Today* **16:**251–253.

Ramaiah, K. D., M. P. Radhamani, K. R. John, D. R. Evans, H. Guyatt, A. Joseph, M. Datta, and P. Vanamail. 2000b. The impact of lymphatic filariasis on labour inputs in southern India: results of a multi-site study. *Ann. Trop. Med. Parasitol.* **94:**353–364.

Ramzy, R. M. R., M. El Setouly, H. Helmy, E. S. Ahmed, K. M. Abad Elaziz, H. A. Farid, W. D. Shannon, and G. J. Weil. 2006. Effect of yearly mass drug administration with diethylcarbamazine and albendazole on bancroftian filariasis in Egypt: a comprehensive assessment. *Lancet* **367:**992–999.

Raso, G., A. Luginbuhl, C. Adjoua, N. T. Tian-Bi, K. D. Silue, B. Matthys, P. Vounatsou, Y. Wang, M. E. Dumas, E. Homes, B. H. Singer, M. Tanner, E. K. N'Goran, and J. Utzinger. 2004. Multiple parasite infections and their relationship to self-reported morbidity in a community of rural Cote d'Ivoire. *Int. J. Epidemiol.* **33:**1092–1102.

Raso, G., J. Utzinger, K. D. Silue, M. Ouattara, A. Yapi, A. Toty, B. Matthys, P. Vounatsou, M. Tanner, and E. K. N'Goran. 2005. Disparities in parasitic infections, perceived ill health and access to health care among poorer and less poor schoolchildren of rural Cote d'Ivoire. *Trop. Med. Int. Health* **10:**42–57.

Raso, G., P. Vounatsou, B. H. Singer, E. N'Goran, M. Tanner, and J. Utzinger. 2006. An integrated approach for risk profiling and spatial prediction of *Schistosoma mansoni*-hookworm coinfection. *Proc. Natl. Acad. Sci. USA* **103:**6934–6939.

Rausch, R. L. 2003. Cystic echinococcosis in the Arctic and Sub-Arctic. *Parasitology* **127:**S73–S85.

Rearwin, D. T., J. H. Tang, and J. W. Hughes. 1997. Causes of blindness among Navajo Indians: an update. *J. Am. Optom. Assoc.* **68:**511–517.

Rebollar-Tellez, E. A., E. Tun-Ku, P. C. Manrique-Saide, and F. J. Andrade-Narvaez. 2005. Relative abundances of sandfly species (Diptera: Phlebotominae) in two villages in the same area of Campeche, in southern Mexico. *Ann. Trop. Med. Parasitol.* **99:**193–201.

Renslo, A. R., and J. H. McKerrow. 2006. Drug discovery and development for neglected parasitic diseases. *Nat. Chem. Biol.* **2:**701–710.

Ribeiro-dos-Santos, G., S. Verjovski-Almeida, and L. C. Leite. 2006. Schistosomiasis—a century searching for chemotherapeutic drugs. *Parasitol. Res.* **99:**505–521.

Riethmiller, S. 2005. From atoxyl to salvarasan: searching for the magic bullet. *Chemotherapy* **51:**234–242.

Rinaldi, A. 2005. The global campaign to eliminate leprosy. *PLoS Med.* **2:**e341.

Ritmeijer, K., and R. N. Davidson. 2003. Royal Society of Tropical Medicine and Hygiene joint meeting with Médecins Sans Frontières at Manson House, London, 20 March 2003: field research in humanitarian medical programmes. Médecins Sans Frontières interventions against kala-azar in the Sudan, 1989–2003. *Trans. R. Soc. Trop. Med. Hyg.* **97:**609–613.

Ross, A. G., D. Vickers, G. R. Olds, S. M. Shah, and D. P. McManus. 2007. Katayama syndrome. *Lancet Infect. Dis.* **7:**218–224.

Roueché, B. 1986. *The Medical Detectives*, vol. 1, p. 68–86. Washington Square Press, New York, NY.

Ruiz-Tiben, E., and D. R. Hopkins. 2006. Dracunculiasis (Guinea worm disease) eradication. *Adv. Parasitol.* **61:**275–309.

Sá, M. R. 2005. The history of tropical medicine in Brazil: the discovery of *Trypanosoma cruzi* by Carlos Chagas and the German school of protozoology. *Parasitologia* **47:**309–317.

Sachs, J. 2007. Sustainable developments. *Sci. Am.* **296:**33.

Sachs, J. D., and P. J. Hotez. 2006. Fighting tropical diseases. *Science* **311:**1521.

Sakti, H., C. Nokes, W. S. Hertanto, S. Hendratno, A. Hall, D. A. Bundy, and Satoto. 1999. Evidence for an association between hookworm infection and cognitive function in Indonesian school children. *Trop. Med. Int. Health* **4:**322–334.

Sargent, R. G., B. W. Dudley, A. S. Fox, and E. J. Lease. 1972. Intestinal helminths in coastal South Carolina: a problem in southeastern United States. *South. Med. J.* **65:**294–298.

Savioli, L., D. Bundy, and A. Tomkins. 1992. Intestinal parasitic infections: a soluble public health problem. *Trans. R. Soc. Trop. Med. Hyg.* **86:**353–354.

Schantz, P. M., and V. C. W. Tsang. 2003. The US Centers for Disease Control and Prevention (CDC) and research and control of cysticercosis. *Acta Tropica* **87:**161–163.

Schneider, M., and M. Moodie. 2002. The destabilizing impacts of HIV/AIDS. Center for Strategic and International Studies, Washington, DC. http://www.kaisernetwork. org/health_cast/uploaded_files/Destabilizing_Impacts_of_AIDS.pdf. Accessed 9 February 2008.

Schofield, C. J., J. Jannin, and R. Salvatella. 2006. The future of Chagas disease control. *Trends Parasitol.* **22:**583–588.

Schwab, A. E., D. A. Boakye, D. Kyelem, and R. K. Prichard. 2005. Detection of benzimidazole resistance-associated mutations in the filarial nematode *Wuchereria bancrofti* and evidence for selection by albendazole and ivermectin combination treatment. *Am. J. Trop. Med. Hyg.* **73:**234–238.

Schwab, A. E., T. S. Churcher, A. J. Schwab, M. G. Basanez, and R. K. Prichard. 2007. An analysis of the population genetics of potential multi-drug resistance in *Wuchereria bancrofti* due to combination chemotherapy. *Parasitology* **134:**1025–1040.

Scollard, D. M., L. B. Adams, T. P. Gillis, J. L. Krahenbuhl, R. W. Truman, and D. L. Williams. 2006. The continuing challenges of leprosy. *Clin. Microbiol. Rev.* **19:**338–381.

Scott, G., and T. J. Coleman. 2002. Leptospirosis, p. 1165–1171. *In* G. C. Cook and A. I. Zumla (ed.), *Manson's Tropical Diseases*, 21st ed. W. B. Saunders, New York, NY.

Secor, W. E. 2006. Interactions between schistosomiasis and infection with HIV-1. *Parasite Immunol.* **28:**597–603.

Sharghi, N., P. Schantz, and P. J. Hotez. 2000. Toxocariasis: an occult cause of childhood neuropsychological deficits and asthma? *Semin. Pediatr. Infect. Dis.* **11:**257–260.

Sharghi, N., P. M. Schantz, L. Caramico, K. Ballas, B. A. Teague, and P. J. Hotez. 2001. Environmental exposure to Toxocara as a possible risk factor for asthma: a clinic-based case-control study. *Clin. Infect. Dis.* **32:**e111–e116.

Sherman, I. W. 2006. *The Power of Plagues.* ASM Press, Washington, DC.

Shuhua, X., P. J. Hotez, and M. Tanner. 2000. Artemether, an effective new agent for chemoprophylaxis against schistosomiasis in China: its in vivo effect on the biochemical metabolism of the Asian schistosome. *Southeast Asian J. Trop. Med. Public Health* **31:**724–732.

Siddiqui, A. A., and S. L. Berk. 2001. Diagnosis of Strongyloides stercoralis infection. *Clin. Infect. Dis.* **33:**1040–1047.

Silva, M. T., F. Portaels, and J. Pedrosa. 2007. Aquatic insects and Mycobacterium ulcerans: an association relevant to Buruli ulcer control? *PLoS Med.* **4:**e63.

Simonsen, P. E. 2002. Filariases, p. 1487–1526. *In* G. C. Cook and A. I. Zumla (ed.), *Manson's Tropical Diseases*, 21st ed. W. B. Saunders, New York, NY.

Sizaire, V., F. Nackers, E. Comte, and F. Portaels. 2006. *Mycobacterium ulcerans* infection: control, diagnosis, and treatment. *Lancet Infect. Dis.* **6:**288–296.

Skolnik, R. 2007. *Essentials of Global Health*, p. 191. Jones and Bartlett Publishers, Sudbury, MA.

Sorvillo, F. J., C. DeGiorgio, and S. H. Waterman. 2007. Deaths from cysticercosis, United States. *Emerg. Infect. Dis.* **13:**230–235.

Stanghellini, A., and T. Josenando. 2001. The situation of sleeping sickness in Angola: a calamity. *Trop. Med. Int. Health* **6:**330–334.

Steinmann, P., J. Keiser, R. Bos, M. Tanner, and J. Utzinger. 2006. Schistosomiasis and water resources development: systematic review, meta-analysis, and estimates of people at risk. *Lancet Infect. Dis.* **6:**411–425.

Stienstra, Y., W. T. van der Graaf, K. Asamoa, and T. S. van der Werf. 2002. Beliefs and attitudes toward Buruli ulcer in Ghana. *Am. J. Trop. Med. Hyg.* **67:**207–213.

Stinear, T. P., A. Mve-Obiang, P. L. Small, W. Frigui, M. J. Pryor, R. Brosch, G. A. Jenkin, P. D. Johnson, J. K. Davies, R. E. Lee, S. Adusumilli, T. Garnier, S. F. Haydock, P. F. Leadlay, and S. T. Cole. 2004. Giant plasmid-encoded polyketide synthases produce the macrolide toxin of *Mycobacterium ulcerans*. *Proc. Natl. Acad. Sci. USA* **101:**1345–1349.

Stoll, N. 1962. On endemic hookworm, where do we stand today? *Exp. Parasitol.* **12:**241–252.

Stoltzfus, R. J., H. M. Chwaya, J. M. Tielsch, K. J. Schulze, M. Albonico, and L. Savioli. 1997a. Epidemiology of iron deficiency anemia in Zanzibari schoolchildren: the importance of hookworms. *Am. J. Clin. Nutr.* **65:**153–159.

Stoltzfus, R. J., M. Dreyfuss, M. P. H. Hababuu, H. M. Chwaya, and M. Albonico. 1997b. Hookworm control as a strategy to prevent iron deficiency. *Nutr. Rev.* **55:**223–232.

Sudarshan, M. K. 2005. Assessing burden of rabies in India: WHO sponsored national multicentric rabies survey, 2003. *Indian J. Community Med.* **30**(3). http://www.indmedical.com/journals.php?journalid=7&issueid=57&articleid=712&action=article. Accessed 11 February 2008.

Taylor, M. J., C. Bandi, and A. Hoerauf. 2005. *Wolbachia* bacterial endosymbionts of filarial nematodes. *Adv. Parasitol.* **60:**247–286.

Teixeira, A. R., R. J. Nascimento, and N. R. Sturm. 2006a. Evolution and pathology in Chagas disease—a review. *Mem. Inst. Oswaldo Cruz* **101:**463–491.

Teixeira, A. R., N. Nitz, M. C. Guimaro, C. Gomes, and C. A. Santos-Buch. 2006b. Chagas disease. *Postgrad. Med. J.* **82:**788–798.

Teklehaimanot, A., J. D. Sachs, and C. Curtis. 2007. Malaria control needs mass distribution of insecticidal bednets. *Lancet* **369:**2143–2146.

Theodorides, J. 1986. *Histoire de la Rage: Cave Canem*. Masson, Paris, France.

Time Magazine. 1962. Mumu, bye-bye. 3 August 1962. http://www.time.com/time/magazine/article/0,9171, 896445,00.html. Accessed 4 April 2008.

Torlesse, H., and M. Hodges. 2000. Anthelminthic treatment and haemaglobin concentrations during pregnancy. *Lancet* **356:**1083.

Townsend, C. A. 2004. Buruli toxin genes decoded. *Proc. Natl. Acad. Sci. USA* **101:**1116–1117.

Tripathi, R. P., D. Katiyar, N. Dwivedi, B. K. Singh, and J. Pandey. 2006. Recent developments in search of antifilarial agents. *Curr. Med. Chem.* **13:**3319–3334.

Tsutsumi, A., T. Izutsu, A. M. Islam, A. N. Maksuda, H. Kato, and S. Wakai. 2007. The quality of life, mental health, and perceived stigma of leprosy patients in Bangladesh. *Soc. Sci. Med.* **64:**2443–2453.

United Nations Human Settlements Programme. 2003. *The Challenge of Slums: Global Report on Human Settlements 2003.* Earthscan Publications, Ltd., London, United Kingdom.

United Nations Population Fund. 2007. State of the world population 2007: unleashing the potential of urban growth. United Nations Population Fund, New York, NY. http://www.unfpa.org/swp/2007/=english/introduction.html. Accessed 9 February 2008.

U. S. Census Bureau. 2007. Poverty: 2006 highlights. U. S. Census Bureau, Washington, DC. http://www.census.gov/hhes/www/poverty/poverty06/pov06hi.html. Accessed 9 February 2008.

Utzinger, J., and J. Keiser. 2006. Urbanization and tropical health—then and now. *Ann. Trop. Med. Parasitol.* **100:**517–533.

Utzinger, J., S. Xiao, E. K. N'Goran, R. Bergquist, and M. Tanner. 2001. The potential of artemether for the control of schistosomiasis. *Int. J. Parasitol.* **31:**1549–1562.

Utzinger, J., X. N. Zhou, M. G. Chen, and R. Bergquist. 2005. Conquering schistosomiasis in China: the long march. *Acta Tropica* **96:**69–96.

Van der Werf, M. J., S. J. de Vlas, S. Brooker, C. W. Looman, N. J. Nagelkerke, J. D. Habbema, and D. Engels. 2003. Quantification of clinical morbidity associated with schistosome infection in sub-Saharan Africa. *Acta Tropica* **86:**125–139.

Vinetz, J. M., G. E. Glass, C. E. Flexner, P. Mueller, and D. C. Kaslow. 1996. Sporadic urban leptospirosis. *Ann. Intern. Med.* **125:**794–798.

Vlassoff, C., M. Weiss, E. B. L. Ovuga, C. Eneanya, P. T. Nwel, S. S. Babalola, A. K. Awedoba, B. Theophilus, P. Cofie, and P. Shetabi. 2000. Gender and the stigma of onchocercal skin disease in Africa. *Soc. Sci. Med.* **50:**1353–1368.

Wallin, M. T., and J. F. Kurtzke. 2004. Neurocysticercosis in the United States: review of an important emerging problem. *Neurology* **63:**1559–1564.

Wansbrough-Jones, M., and R. Phillips. 2006. Buruli ulcer: emerging from obscurity. *Lancet* **367:**1849–1858.

Warrell, M. J. 2002. Rabies, p. 808–821. *In* G. C. Cook and A. I. Zumla (ed.), *Manson's Tropical Diseases*, 21st ed. W. B. Saunders, New York, NY.

Warrell, M. J., and D. A. Warrell. 2004. Rabies and other lyssavirus diseases. *Lancet* **363:**959–969.

Wei, W.-P. 1958. The people's boundless energy during the current leap forward. I. New victories on the anti-schistosomiasis front. *Chinese Med. J.* **77:**107–111.

Weina, P. J., R. C. Neafie, G. Wortmann, M. Polhemus, and N. E. Aronson. 2004. Old world leishmaniasis: an emerging infection among deployed US military and civilian workers. *Clin. Infect. Dis.* **39:**1674–1680.

Weiss, M. G., and J. Ramakrishna. 2006. Stigma interventions and research for international health. *Lancet* **367:**536–538.

Welbrun, S. C., P. G. Coleman, I. Maudlin, E. M. Fevre, M. Odiit, and M. C. Eisler. 2006. Crisis, what crisis? Control of Rhodesian sleeping sickness. *Trends Parasitol.* **22:**123–128.

White, A. C., Jr., and R. L. Atmar. 2002. Infections in Hispanic immigrants. *Clin. Infect. Dis.* **34:**1627–1632.

WHO Expert Committee on the Control of Chagas Disease. 2002. *Control of Chagas Disease: Second Report of the WHO Expert Committee.* World Health Organization Technical Report Series no. 905. World Health Organization, Geneva, Switzerland.

Wiesel, E. 1978. *A Jew Today*, p. 17. Vintage Books, New York, NY.

Willard, R. J., A. M. Jeffcoat, P. M. Benson, and D. C. Walsh. 2005. Cutaneous leishmaniasis in soldiers from Fort Campbell, Kentucky returning from Operation Iraqi Freedom highlights diagnostic and therapeutic options. *J. Am. Acad. Dermatol.* **52:**977–987.

Williamson, A. L., P. Lecchi, B. E. Turk, Y. Choe, P. J. Hotez, J. H. McKerrow, L. C. Cantley, M. Sajid, and A. Loukas. 2004. A multi-enzyme cascade of hemoglobin proteolysis in the intestine of blood-feeding hookworms. *J. Biol. Chem.* **279:**3590–3597.

Wilson, J. F., R. L. Rausch, and F. R. Wilson. 1995. Alveolar hydatid disease. *Ann. Surg.* **221:**315–323.

World Bank. 2003. School deworming at a glance. World Bank, Washington, DC. http://siteresources.worldbank.org/INTPHAAG/Resources/AAGDewormingEng110603.pdf. Accessed 9 February 2008.

World Health Organization. 2003. Neglected diseases that disable millions, p. 104–153. *In* M. K. Kindhauser (ed.), *Communicable Diseases 2002: Global Defence against the Infectious Disease Threat.* World Health Organization, Geneva, Switzerland.

World Health Organization. 2006a. Global Programme to Eliminate Lymphatic Filariasis. *Wkly. Epidemiol. Rec.* **22:**221–232.

World Health Organization. 2006b. *Neglected Tropical Diseases: Hidden Successes, Emerging Opportunities.* World Health Organization, Geneva, Switzerland.

World Health Organization. 2006c. Onchocerciasis (river blindness). *Wkly. Epidemiol. Rec.* **81:**293–296.

World Health Organization. 2006d. *Preventive Chemotherapy in Human Helminthiasis.* World Health Organization, Geneva, Switzerland.

World Health Organization. 2007. Tuberculosis. World Health Organization, Geneva, Switzerland. http://www.who.int/mediacentre/factsheets/fs104/en/. Accessed 9 February 2008.

World Health Organization. 2008a. Dengue/dengue haemorrhagic fever. World Health Organization, Geneva, Switzerland. http://www.who.int/csr/disease/dengue/en. Accessed 9 February 2008.

World Health Organization. 2008b. Rabies. World Health Organization, Geneva, Switzerland. http://www.who.int/immunization/topics/rabies/en/index.html. Accessed 9 February 2008.

World Health Organization. 2008c. Leprosy today. World Health Organization, Geneva, Switzerland. http://www.who.int/lep/en/index.html. Accessed 9 February 2008.

World Health Organization. 2008d. Onchocerciasis Elimination Program for the Americas (OEPA). World Health Organization, Geneva, Switzerland. http://www.who.int/blindness/partnerships/onchocerciasis_oepa/en/index.html. Accessed 9 February 2008.

World Health Organization. 2008e. Pursue high-quality DOTS expansion and enhancement. World Health Organization, Geneva, Switzerland. http://www.who.int/tb/dots/en/. Accessed 9 February 2008.

World Health Organization. 2008f. Prevention of blindness and visual impairment. World Health Organization, Geneva, Switzerland. http://www.who.int/blindness/en/. Accessed 9 February 2008.

World Health Organization. 2008g. Historical background and important dates. World Health Organization, Geneva, Switzerland. http://www.who.int/dracunculiasis/background/en/index.html. Accessed 9 February 2008.

World Health Organization. 2008h. Dengue and dengue haemorrhagic fever. World Health Organization, Geneva, Switzerland. http://www.who.int/mediacentre/factsheets/fs117/en/. Accessed 9 February 2008.

World Health Organization. 1995. Expert committee on onchocerciasis control. Technical report series no. 852. World Health Organization, Geneva, Switzerland.

Wright, J. W. (ed.). 2006. *The 2006 New York Times Almanac.* Penguin, New York, NY.

Wyatt, J. 2007. Rabies—update on a global disease. *Pediatr. Infect. Dis. J.* **26:**351–352.

Xiao, S. H., W. Hui-Ming, M. Tanner, J. Utzinger, and W. Chong. 2005. Tribendimidine: a promising, safe and broad-spectrum anthelmintic agent from China. *Acta Tropica* **94:**1–14.

Yamagata, Y., and J. Nakagawa. 2006. Control of Chagas disease. *Adv. Parasitol.* **61:**129–165.

Zhong, C., and T. Zhen. 1991. Control and surveillance of filariasis in Shandong. *Chin. Med. J.* **104:**179–185.

Zijlstra, E. E., and A. M. El-Hassan. 2001. Leishmaniasis in Sudan. 3. Visceral leishmaniasis. *Trans. R. Soc. Trop. Med. Hyg.* **95**(Suppl. 1):S1/27–S1/58.

Zimmermann, M. B., and R. Hurrell. 2007. Nutritional iron deficiency. *Lancet* **370:**511–520.

Index